The Homeopathic Book

Dr Víctor Denis Purcell

Published by Dr Víctor Denis Purcell, 2023.

While every precaution has been taken in the preparation of this book, the publisher assumes no responsibility for errors or omissions, or for damages resulting from the use of the information contained herein.

THE HOMEOPATHIC BOOK

First edition. December 2, 2023.

Copyright © 2023 Dr Víctor Denis Purcell.

ISBN: 979-8223298984

Written by Dr Víctor Denis Purcell.

Homeopathy, holistic healing, remedies, natural medicine, astrology, patient tendencies, gender-specific health, Materia Medica, ancient practices, modern applications, healing principles, remedy selection, mind-body connection, individualized treatment, Samuel Hahnemann, dilution, intrinsic healing, practical applications, men's health, women's health, astrological inquiry, foundational principles, homeopathic integration, transformative wellness, emotional constitution, physical symptoms, spiritual alignment, comprehensive insights, alternative medicine, therapeutic journey.

The Homeopathic Book

Homeopathy: An In-depth Exploration of Healing Principles and Practices

This book delves deep into homeopathic medicine, shedding light on its foundational principles, rich history, and evolving philosophy. Starting from its inception by Samuel Hahnemann, readers are introduced to the core concept of "like cures like," exploring the use of minutely diluted remedies that harness the body's intrinsic healing capabilities. The book further elucidates vital homeopathic tenets, such as the principle of minimal dosage and the direction of cure, which help monitor and guide the healing journey.

A notable aspect of homeopathy is its holistic approach, emphasizing the importance of comprehensive case-taking. Through keen observation, active listening, and detailed questioning, practitioners piece together the patient's physical, emotional, and mental state, ensuring the selection of a remedy that resonates with their unique symptom picture.

Exploring the Materia Medica introduces readers to various homeopathic remedies derived from nature, explaining their unique properties and indications. The book also extends its focus to practical applications, demonstrating homeopathy's efficacy in addressing minor first-aid conditions and specific health concerns related to men and women.

In a blend of ancient wisdom and modern practices, the intriguing integration of astrology in case-taking is discussed, offering more profound insights into a patient's constitution and aiding in remedy selection.

As we navigate towards a future where integrative medicine gains prominence, this book discusses the burgeoning prospects of homeopathy, highlighting its increasing acceptance in mainstream healthcare and the promising research avenues that beckon. This comprehensive guide provides both a foundation and a visionary outlook, encapsulating the timeless essence and evolving dynamism of homeopathic medicine.

Disclaimer

Please read the following terms and conditions carefully before proceeding.

General Information Purposes Only: The information provided in the following is for general informational and entertainment purposes only. All information is provided in good faith; however, the author makes no representation or warranty of any kind, express or implied, regarding the accuracy, adequacy, validity, reliability, availability, or completeness of any information on the following.

Not Medical Advice: The content provided below is not intended to be a substitute for professional medical advice, diagnosis, or treatment. Always seek the advice of your physician or other qualified health providers with any questions you may have regarding a medical condition or health concerns.

No Doctor-Patient Relationship: reading the

information below does not constitute establishing a doctor-patient relationship. Any health information communicated is not an endorsement, diagnosis, or treatment regimen.

Professional Assistance: You must not rely on the information below as an alternative to medical advice from your doctor or other professional healthcare providers. If you believe you are experiencing any medical condition, seek immediate medical attention from a licensed healthcare provider.

Risks of Self-Diagnosis: Self-diagnosis can lead to harm, and healthcare professionals must perform diagnosis and treatment.

Limitation of Warranties: The medical information provided is "as is" without any representations or warranties, express or implied. The author makes no representations or warranties concerning the medical report.

Liability: You agree to release the offer from all liability and to hold him harmless from any legal claims related to the medical information provided.

Contact a Doctor: Do not disregard, avoid, or delay obtaining medical advice from a qualified healthcare provider because of something you may have read in this book or below.

You do understand and agree to the terms of this disclaimer. If you do not agree with these terms, you are not authorized to obtain information from or otherwise proceed.

Chapters headings

Chapter 1: Introduction to homeopathic medicine

Chapter 2: Materia Medica

Chapter 3: Homeopathic medicine for men's and women's health

Chapter 4: Homeopathy for First Aid Conditions

Chapter 5: The use of astrology in case-taking

Chapter 6: Prospects of homeopathic medicine, and a summary of information.

Chapter 1: Introduction to homeopathic medicine

In this opening chapter, we delve into the fundamental principles, history, and philosophy that formed the backbone of homeopathic medicine. We explore the core concepts of "like cures like" and the use of highly diluted remedies to stimulate the body's healing responses and innate wisdom. Additionally, we journey through the rich historical roots of homeopathy, from its inception by Samuel Hahnemann to the development and evolution of his principles over time. By understanding its foundation, readers will understand the principles underlining this evolved form of medicine.

The Genesis of Homeopathy: Samuel Hahnemann's Vision

The story of homeopathy begins with the work of a German physician, Samuel Hahnemann, in the late 18th century. Disillusioned by the medical practices of his time, which he saw as barbaric and ineffective, Hahnemann sought a more humane and rational approach to healing. His relentless pursuit for a better method led him to discover the principle he called similia similibus curentur, or "like cures like," which became the cornerstone of homeopathic medicine. This was a radical departure from the conventional medical practices of bloodletting, purging, and the use of toxic substances. Hahnemann's vision was for a medical system that supported the body's natural tendency to heal itself, a principle he found echoed in ancient texts, but until then, not rigorously applied or understood in the context of a comprehensive medical system.

The Law of Similars: Understanding "Like Cures Like"

"Like cures like," the foundational principle of homeopathy, posits that substances capable of causing disease symptoms in healthy individuals can treat similar symptoms in the sick. Hahnemann came upon this idea while translating a medical text and took particular interest in a claim regarding using cinchona bark (from which quinine is derived) for treating malaria. Experimenting on himself, he ingested cinchona and noted it produced symptoms reminiscent of malaria. This observation was the catalyst for his principle, leading to further experimentation and the development of a doctrine that proposed that by using these similar symptoms as a guide, a physician could select substances that would stimulate the body's innate healing processes. This law not only signified a shift in the understanding of treatment but also suggested a profound interconnectedness between humans and nature—a relationship that homeopathy seeks to harness.

As Hahnemann continued his experiments, he began documenting the specific effects of various substances on healthy individuals, a process he termed "provings." During these provings, volunteers, including Hahnemann himself, would take a sense to record the detailed physical, emotional, and mental symptoms that resulted. These observations were meticulously cataloged, creating the first rudimentary materia medica of homeopathy. This compendium of remedies, along with their corresponding symptom profiles, became a critical guide for treatment, allowing homeopaths to match a patient's symptom picture with a precise remedy.

Through continued practice and experimentation, Hahnemann refined the process of preparing homeopathic remedies. He introduced the method of potentization, which involves systematically diluting the original substance and succussing (vigorously shaking) it at each dilution step. Hahnemann proposed that this process not only reduced the toxicity of the actual substance but also enhanced its curative powers. The notion was that even when diluted beyond the point of containing any molecules of the original substance, the remedy would retain an imprint or 'memory' of the substance's healing properties.

The concept of individualized treatment is another pivotal element of homeopathy. In stark contrast to the one-size-fits-all approach of conventional medicine of the time, homeopathy insisted on the uniqueness of each patient's experience of illness. Hahnemann argued that effective treatment could not be achieved without thoroughly understanding the patient's symptoms, lifestyle, and psychological state. This holistic view acknowledges the complexity of human health and places significant emphasis on tailoring the remedy to the person, not just the disease.

The holistic approach extended beyond the physical symptoms to include emotional and mental aspects of health, an idea that was innovative for Hahnemann's time. He observed that emotional states such as grief or shock could have a profound impact on physical fitness and should, therefore, be considered in treatment. This perspective was a departure from the mainstream medical thought of the era, which primarily focused on the physical body and often ignored the mental and emotional components of illness.

Hahnemann's development of homeopathy also brought about a different perspective on disease. He saw disease as a disturbance of the body's vital force—an energetic principle maintaining health. Homeopathic remedies, therefore, were believed to work by stimulating the body's intense energy to restore balance and health. This vitalistic view of medicine was met with both interest and skepticism, as it challenged the emerging mechanistic views of the body that were gaining traction in scientific circles.

The practice of homeopathy began to spread as Hahnemann's students and followers continued to practice and teach his methods. By the early 19th century, homeopathy had started to take root in Europe and America. It offered a stark contrast to the often harsh and invasive medical practices of the time, contributing to its popularity. Homeopathy's promise of gentle, non-toxic treatments appealed to patients who had grown weary of conventional medicine's more damaging remedies.

The global spread of homeopathy was met with varied receptions. In some countries, it integrated well with existing medical systems, while in others, it was met with resistance from the established medical community. Despite this, by the mid-19th century, homeopathy had become increasingly popular, with numerous homeopathic hospitals, colleges, and pharmacies based across Europe and the United States. This period is often considered the golden age of homeopathy, with its practices widely embraced by physicians and the public.

Despite its growth and popularity, homeopathy's principles were not without controversy. The idea of potentization, in particular, drew criticism for its departure from the principles of chemistry and physics. The high dilutions used in homeopathy, often beyond where any molecule of the original substance remains, became a focal point for debate. Critics argued that any benefit felt by patients was due to the placebo effect rather than any physiological impact of the homeopathic remedy.

In response to the skepticism, homeopaths pointed to the empirical nature of their practice, emphasizing the clinical outcomes and the recoveries they witnessed. They argued that homeopathy's efficacy could not be denied simply because it did not fit within the current scientific paradigms. The debate over homeopathy's legitimacy has continued into the modern era, embodying the tension between empirical experience and the demand for evidence-based medicine.

The homeopathic community has also engaged in ongoing research to explore and validate the mechanisms behind their remedies. Efforts to scientifically investigate homeopathy have included clinical trials, observational studies, and laboratory research. Despite the challenges presented by homeopathic principles to conventional scientific methodologies, proponents continue to seek ways to understand how the dilute substances in homeopathy might interact with the body's processes. This research is part of a broader attempt to bridge the gap between homeopathy and mainstream medicine, fostering a dialogue that could lead to a more integrative approach to health care, where the insights of homeopathy are considered alongside those of conventional medicine. The quest for a deeper understanding of homeopathy thus reflects a more significant movement towards an inclusive knowledge of healing and medicine, one that acknowledges the value of diverse medical traditions and the complexity of human health.

Stop

The Law of Similars: Understanding "Like Cures Like"

Embarking on a radical departure from conventional medical thinking, the Law of Similars forms the bedrock of homeopathic medicine. This concept, envisioned by Samuel Hahnemann, asserts that a disease can be cured by a substance that produces similar symptoms in healthy people. It is this paradoxical idea that underpins all homeopathic remedies and treatments. Hahnemann's insight into the Law of Similars did not arise from mysticism or conjecture but from a disciplined and meticulous method of inquiry and observation. He began by self-administering substances and recording the effects they produced, thus laying the groundwork for a systematic approach to healing that was both consistent and reproducible.

The principle of "like cures like" offered a sharp contrast to the medical paradigms of the 18th century, which often involved treating opposites with opposites. Instead of using compounds that would counteract symptoms, Hahnemann's method sought to mirror the disease process, thereby stimulating the body's natural defenses. This approach hinged on a deep understanding of symptoms not merely as manifestations of disease but as reflections of the body's attempts to heal itself.

Hahnemann's systematic approach to discovering the Law of Similars was rigorous. He engaged in what would now be termed clinical trials, though rudimentary, to test his theory. By documenting the reactions of healthy individuals to various substances, he built a database of symptoms and associated substances that could induce them. This exhaustive compilation allowed for a reference point from which remedies could be prescribed with precision, respecting the nuances of individual patients' experiences of illness.

As homeopathy grew, so did the practice of documenting "provings." These provings were detailed examinations and recordings of the symptoms induced by substances in a group of healthy volunteers. The precision with which these symptoms were recorded underscored the meticulous nature of the homeopathic practice. Each proof was added to the expanding knowledge repository, helping homeopaths match a patient's symptom profile with a specific remedy shown to produce a similar profile in healthy individuals.

Refining the Law of Similars necessitated a balance between specificity and generalization. While Hahnemann's principle dictated that the remedy should be similar to the disease, there was also an understanding that each person's experience of symptoms was unique. The subtleties of a patient's emotional and physical state were to be carefully considered, ensuring that the chosen remedy addressed the disease in its full personal context.

Applying the Law of Similars in practice also implied an individualized dosage. Hahnemann knew that the same substance could cause different reactions in different people or even in the same person under other conditions. Therefore, determining the right potency and dosage was as crucial as selecting the correct substance. This personalized approach was a significant departure from the one-size-fits-all mentality prevalent in mainstream medicine at the time.

The therapeutic implications of the Law of Similars extended beyond mere symptom relief. In homeopathy, the aim was not just to alleviate symptoms but to address the underlying disturbance in the vital force. By selecting a remedy that mirrored the patient's complete symptom picture, homeopaths believed they could prompt a more profound, more curative response, engaging the body's inherent self-healing capabilities.

Critics of homeopathy often targeted the Law of Similars, labeling it as scientifically implausible. The argument was that the principle did not align with the emerging biomedical model, which was grounded in the identification and direct antagonism of pathogenic factors. Homeopathy, with its reliance on symptom similarity rather than pathogen opposition, was often dismissed as unscientific by the standards of the day.

In defense, homeopaths pointed to the empirical nature of their work. They argued that the Law of Similars was derived from observation and experiment, hallmarks of the scientific method. The efficacy of a remedy, in their view, was validated by the observable improvement in the patient's condition following its administration, regardless of the prevailing medical theories of the time.

The debate around the Law of Similars underscores a broader philosophical question about the nature of healing and the role of medicine. Homeopathy posits a vision of treatment that is attuned to the subtleties of the individual and the nuanced expression of disease, inviting a more personalized and holistic approach to health. Despite the skepticism it faces, the Law of Similars continues to inspire those who seek an alternative to conventional medicine's sometimes impersonal and reductionist approach.

The Art of Dilution: Potentization and Succussion

In the intricate practice of homeopathy, potentization and succussion are pivotal processes that transform substances into therapeutic agents. Potentization involves diluting the original substance systematically, often to a point where no molecules of the starting material are detectable, following the homeopathic belief in the strength of highly diluted preparations. Succussion, the act of vigorously shaking the substance at each stage of dilution, is believed to transfer the essence or 'energy' of the meaning into the medium, typically water or alcohol. Hahnemann, who was very much an empiricist, developed these methods to mitigate the toxic effects he observed when administering undiluted substances. He discovered that although the physical presence of the original importance diminished, its healing properties not only persisted but seemed enhanced.

This methodology stands at the core of homeopathy's departure from conventional pharmacology, which typically relies on dose-dependent effects. The theory behind potentization suggests that the process of diluting and shaking imprints the memory of the substance onto the diluent, which then interacts with the body's vital force. Hahnemann proposed that through this method, the curative properties are retained and amplified without the risk of toxic side effects. This concept challenges the conventional dose-response relationship and has been a subject of intrigue and skepticism within the broader medical community.

Each level of dilution in the potentization process, known as potency, is marked by a specific ratio. Standard potencies such as 6C or 30C indicate the substance has been diluted to 1 part in 100, six, or thirty times over, respectively. The strength selected is tailored to the individual patient and is informed by the nature of their symptoms. Acute symptoms might be treated with lower potencies, while more deep-seated or chronic conditions could be addressed with higher powers. The choice of strength is a critical component of the homeopathic prescription, reflecting the nuanced understanding of the dynamic between the remedy, the patient, and their disease.

Succussion adds another layer to the potentization process. Hahnemann instructed that the mixture should be struck against an elastic body, a procedure he believed vital to activate the medicinal properties of the solution. While mainstream science has yet to elucidate the mechanisms by which succussion could enhance the therapeutic efficacy of a homeopathic solution, practitioners and patients of homeopathy attest to the qualitative difference between succussed and unsuccussed remedies, suggesting that the physical process of shaking is integral to remedy preparation.

The debate on the plausibility of potentization touches upon fundamental principles of chemistry and physics. Skeptics argue that homeopathic dilutions, often beyond Avogadro's number, should theoretically negate any chemical activity of the original substance. Proponents counter that the efficacy of homeopathic remedies is empirically evident and warrants an open-minded investigation into the possibility of non-chemical forms of biological activity. This remains a frontier where homeopathy and conventional science often clash, with each side holding firm to their foundational principles.

Despite the controversy, potentization has remained an essential aspect of homeopathic medicine. It represents a unique intersection between art and science, where the precise methodology is informed by a philosophy that extends beyond the worldly confines of conventional medicinal chemistry. This reflects a broader holistic approach, where the remedy is prepared with intent and understanding of its eventual dynamic interaction with the patient's vital force.

The principles of potentization and succussion also reflect the importance of process in homeopathy. It is not merely the substance that imparts healing but how it is prepared and administered. This highlights a characteristic aspect of homeopathy – the belief in a process-oriented approach to healing, where every step, from remedy selection to preparation, is executed with careful deliberation and purpose.

Homeopathic practitioners uphold that the process of potentization is as much an art as it is a science. It requires not only an understanding of the technical aspects but also an intuitive grasp of the more subtle, energetic shifts that the process entails. The art of potentization, therefore, is a synthesis of empirical methods and holistic insight – a dance between the tangible and the intangible aspects of healing.

The persistent practice and popularity of homeopathy, despite the lack of scientific clarity on potentization and succussion, suggest a resonant efficacy that many find convincing. While this efficacy might not yet be entirely explicable in scientific terms, the empirical results observed by homeopathic practitioners provide a compelling narrative for many patients seeking alternative or complementary treatments.

In conclusion, the practices of potentization and succussion remain central to the identity of homeopathic medicine. They encapsulate the willingness of homeopathy to embrace concepts that challenge the status quo, inviting ongoing dialogue and investigation into the nature of healing and the potential for medicine to operate beyond the boundaries of the measurable substance.

The Principle of the Minimum Dose in homeopathy is the concept that the lowest amount of a substance needed to initiate a healing response is the most desirable dosage. This principle stems from the desire to avoid side effects and the philosophy that the body's natural healing processes should be supported but not overpowered or suppressed by the treatment. Hahnemann, witnessing the harsh methods of conventional treatments of his time, which often included bloodletting and high doses of toxic substances, sought a more gentle and respectful approach to healing. This led to his pioneering work in diminishing quantities to the minimum required to effect change. This practice not only stood in contrast to mainstream medicine but also defined a core tenet of homeopathic philosophy.

The minimum dose principle operates in tandem with potentization to produce remedies that are believed to interact with the body's vital force rather than the physiological body directly. The rationale is that while conventional medicine often focuses on changing physical symptoms through direct chemical action, homeopathy aims to trigger the body's inherent self-regulatory mechanisms. It is thought that even the subtlest introduction of the correct homeopathic remedy can catalyze a profound healing response without overwhelming the body's systems.

Implementing the minimum dose is considered a highly individualized endeavor. Homeopaths spend extensive time understanding a patient's unique symptom profile, history, and constitution before determining the precise remedy and dosage. This specificity ensures that treatment is tailored to the patient, adhering to the belief that the minimum dose is not a fixed quantity but a relative measure, dependent on the individual's sensitivity and the nature of their condition.

In clinical practice, the minimum dose is given just often enough to maintain healing momentum. The homeopath carefully observes the patient's response and adjusts the frequency and potency of doses accordingly. The goal is to provide enough stimulus for the body's healing response without causing aggravation or unnecessary repetition of the remedy. In this way, the principle of the minimum dose respects the body's pace and capacity for recovery.

Critics of homeopathy have often cited the minimum dose as a point of contention, arguing that such minute doses, often beyond the end of molecular presence, cannot possibly have any effect.

Homeopaths, however, assert that clinical outcomes justify their approach and call for an expanded understanding of drug action that encompasses more than just the material dose-response relationship that dominates pharmacology.

Despite skepticism from the broader medical community, homeopathy's principle of the minimum dose has found resonance in areas where there is growing concern over the overuse of medication and its side effects. It presents an alternative that aligns with the modern movement toward more sustainable and conservative use of medical interventions.

The principle of the minimum dose also speaks to a philosophical stance that recognizes the body as a self-healing organism, with medicine's role being to support rather than usurp the healing process. It suggests a partnership between practitioner and patient, where the former provides the stimulus and the latter's body performs the healing work.

Homeopaths also view the minimum dose as a means of honoring the body's wisdom. By using the minor intervention necessary, they believe they acknowledge and respect the body's capacity to correct imbalances and restore health. This starkly contrasts with interventions that seek to control or suppress symptoms without addressing underlying imbalances.

The ongoing use of the minimum dose in homeopathic practice is a testament to the enduring principles upon which homeopathy was founded. It represents a commitment to a form of medicine that is gentle, respectful, and aligned with a holistic view of health. The philosophy underlying the minimum dose continues to challenge the conventional medical model and offers a perspective on healing that is subtle yet, for many, deeply resonant.

In summary, the Principle of the Minimum Dose is integral to homeopathy, emphasizing gentle intervention and respect for the body's inherent healing capabilities. While this principle defies conventional pharmacological wisdom, it remains a cornerstone of homeopathic medicine, embodying a commitment to a less invasive and more patient-centric approach to health care.

The Individualized Approach: The Patient as the Central Focus

The Individualized Approach in homeopathy is a distinctive aspect that views each patient as a unique entity, requiring a tailored treatment strategy. This contrasts with the one-size-fits-all methodology often seen in conventional medicine, where diseases are typically treated with standardized protocols. Homeopaths believe that two individuals presenting with what might be classified as the same illness in traditional terms may need completely different homeopathic remedies. This individualization is based on a comprehensive assessment of the patient's physical, emotional, and mental symptoms, along with their personal medical history and life circumstances.

This patient-centered focus demands a thorough case-taking process, one of the most time-intensive parts of homeopathic practice. Homeopaths conduct in-depth interviews to gain insights into the patient's subtle symptoms and responses to various influences, including environmental factors and stressors. The detailed questioning can explore aspects such as food preferences, sleep patterns, and emotional temperament, which might not seem directly related to the illness but are considered crucial in selecting the most fitting remedy.

The homeopathic repertory, an extensive index of symptoms and their associated remedies, is a crucial tool for individualizing treatment. By matching the patient's unique symptom profile with the nuanced details in the repertory, homeopaths can pinpoint remedies that correspond most closely to the patient's condition. This process, referred to as 'repertorization,' reflects the intricate nature of remedy selection and the high degree of customization involved in homeopathic treatment.

This individualized approach acknowledges the complexity of the human condition, respecting that the manifestations of illness are as diverse as the people who experience them. It operates on the premise that effective treatment must not only address the disease but must also resonate with the patient's overall well-being. This level of customization is designed to stimulate the body's healing processes in a way most aligned with the individual's vitality and health.

Homeopaths view the individualization of treatment as a way to honor the whole person rather than merely focusing on isolated symptoms or diseases. This holistic view extends to understanding and treating the patient's mental and emotional health as integral components of overall well-being. By doing so, homeopathy seeks not only to alleviate symptoms but also to enhance the patient's overall vitality and capacity for self-healing.

The individualized approach also reflects the adaptability of homeopathic treatment. As patients undergo therapy and their conditions evolve, their treatment plans are reassessed and adjusted accordingly. This dynamic process is responsive to changes in the patient's symptoms and health status, allowing for a flexible and responsive treatment strategy that evolves.

Homeopathy's emphasis on the individual has been praised for its compassionate, patient-centered care and criticized for its lack of standardized treatment protocols. Yet, despite differing opinions, the approach has remained a hallmark of the practice, signifying the depth and attention given to each patient's unique experience of illness.

The individualized approach of homeopathy also underlines the relationship between patient and practitioner, fostering a partnership built on mutual trust and in-depth understanding. The homeopath's role is as much a listener and interpreter as a healer, and aspect patients often find reassuring and empowering.

This bespoke approach to medicine particularly appeals to those who feel marginalized or misunderstood by conventional healthcare systems. It often attracts patients seeking a more personalized and empathetic approach to their health concerns and who are willing to engage actively in their journey toward health.

In summary, the homeopathic practitioner places the patient at the center of the treatment process, emphasizing a tailored strategy that respects the complexity and individuality of each person. It is a meticulous practice that seeks to understand the patient, providing a customized treatment plan designed to work in harmony with the body's natural healing abilities.

The Holistic Philosophy in homeopathy embodies the principle of treating the individual in their entirety, not just the isolated symptoms of a disease. This approach is foundational to homeopathic medicine, reflecting a deep respect for the complex interplay between mind, body, and spirit in the pursuit of health and healing. It is based on the understanding that symptoms are expressions of the body's attempt to heal itself and that true healing involves restoring balance within the whole person.

In homeopathic practice, this philosophy involves meticulously considering the patient's physical symptoms, emotional state, mental health, and overall life circumstances. The holistic approach recognizes that emotional disturbances or life stressors can manifest as physical ailments and vice versa. Homeopaths, therefore, give weight to psychological well-being and emotional balance as integral to the health of the body, taking into account factors like personal relationships, life stress, and mental outlook.

This comprehensive view extends to the patient's physical examination, which includes an evaluation of their general vitality and susceptibilities. It is not uncommon for a homeopath to inquire about a patient's energy levels, sleep quality, and even dreams, as all are considered relevant to the person's holistic health profile. The premise is that any imbalance or disharmony in one part of the system can influence the whole, hence the importance of a thorough and inclusive assessment.

By addressing the person as a whole, homeopathy aims to bring about a state of harmony where health can flourish on all levels. The remedies selected are intended to support the body's self-healing mechanisms, encouraging a return to a state of balance rather than merely suppressing symptoms. Homeopaths believe that when the body is in balance, symptoms resolve as a natural consequence.

The holistic philosophy also considers patients' perceptions and experiences of their illness as valuable diagnostic tools. Homeopaths listen carefully to how patients describe their symptoms, recognizing that the words and images people choose can provide insight into their inner state and help guide the selection of an appropriate remedy.

This philosophical stance is particularly relevant in chronic illnesses, where symptoms can be complex and multifaceted. Homeopathy's holistic approach seeks to understand the underlying patterns that sustain illness, working towards a more sustainable and long-term restoration of health rather than a quick fix of symptoms.

The homeopathic consultation is a holistic exercise, often resembling a therapeutic dialogue. The safe and open environment provided during the consultation is considered a part of the healing process, as it allows patients to express themselves fully and to be heard without judgment.

The holistic approach reflects a broader shift in health consciousness that values wellness over the mere absence of disease. It aligns with preventative health measures and lifestyle changes that support overall well-being—homeopaths often counsel patients on diet, exercise, and mindfulness practices, which complement the remedies provided.

In a world where health care can often be fragmented and compartmentalized, homeopathy's holistic philosophy offers a more integrated and person-centered approach. It appeals to individuals seeking a form of medicine that acknowledges the complexities of their experience and the interconnectedness of their symptoms.

In summary, the Holistic Philosophy in homeopathy is about recognizing and treating the multifaceted nature of individuals, aiming to restore balance on all levels of being. It is an approach that underscores the uniqueness of each healing journey, prioritizing personalized care and the understanding that health is a state of complete physical, mental, and social well-being.

The Dynamis Concept: Vital Force as the Essence of Life

This concept, in homeopathy, also known as the vital force or vital energy, is fundamental to its understanding of health and disease. It posits that a dynamic energy force animates all living beings, governing their physical functions and adaptive processes. In homeopathy, this vital force maintains equilibrium and, when imbalanced, leads to symptoms of illness. The role of homeopathic remedies, then, is to stimulate the necessary energy to restore balance and health.

This vitalist perspective differentiates homeopathy from many other forms of medicine, incredibly conventional Western medicine, which is mainly mechanical and biochemical in its approach. Homeopaths assert that the vital force, although not directly observable, is discernible by the effects it produces — much like the movement of the leaves knows the wind. The state of the vital force is reflected in the individual's overall well-being, including their mental, emotional, and physical conditions.

In practice, when a homeopath selects a remedy, they seek to match the remedy's energy with the energy of the patient's disturbed vital force. It is believed that the remedy's dynamic quality, enhanced through the process of potentization, interacts with the essential power, providing the impetus for the self-healing process to commence. This is why minute doses are sufficient; it is the energy or 'information' of the remedy, rather than a material quantity, that is key.

The concept of vital force as the driver of health leads to the holistic treatment of patients. Homeopaths view symptoms as expressions of a disturbed essential force and hence do not aim to suppress them but rather to understand what they indicate about the underlying imbalance. This perspective values symptoms as critical guides to selecting an appropriate remedy rather than as nuisances to be eliminated.

The particular force is also central to the homeopathic understanding of disease progression. Disease is seen not merely as a specific organ or system dysfunction but as a more profound disturbance of the vital force. Thus, treatment success is measured by an improvement in the patient's overall vitality and a return to a sense of well-being rather than just the disappearance of particular symptoms.

The vital force concept resonates with several traditional healing systems, which also recognize an invisible life force — such as qi in Traditional Chinese Medicine or prana in Ayurveda. This cross-cultural recognition of life energy that must be balanced for good health is a point of connection between homeopathy and other holistic health practices.

Various factors, including emotional states, environmental conditions, and lifestyle choices, influence the strength and harmony of the vital force. Therefore, a homeopath may guide diet, stress management, and other aspects of life that can support the patient's vitality. It's understood that maintaining a solid and balanced vital force is critical to resilience against illness.

In dealing with chronic diseases, the concept of the Dynamis is particularly significant. Homeopaths consider the long-term vitality and energy patterns of the individual, aiming to gradually restore the disturbed vital force to a state of equilibrium. Chronic symptoms indicate a deep-seated imbalance in the strong influence that requires a sustained therapeutic strategy.

The vital force also informs the homeopathic perspective on prevention. A well-balanced essential energy confers immunity and resilience, reducing disease susceptibility. Thus, homeopathy places a strong emphasis on strengthening the vital force as a means of preventing illness and promoting long-term health.

In summary, the vital force concept is a cornerstone of homeopathic medicine, representing the essential energy that, when in balance, leads to health and, when disturbed, results in disease. Homeopathic treatment is designed to work with this vital force, aiding the body's inherent ability to heal itself and maintain equilibrium. This notion of an animating energy unique to each individual is central to homeopathy's individualized and holistic approach to health and healing.

The Principle of Potentization: Unlocking Remedial Energy

The Principle of Potentization is a hallmark of homeopathic medicine, representing a unique process by which remedies are prepared to enhance their healing properties. This involves serial dilution and succussion (vigorous shaking) of a substance, intending to release its energetic potential. Homeopaths believe that through this process, the remedy becomes more effective by stimulating the body's vital force more powerfully while minimizing the risk of toxic side effects.

Potentization is rooted in the idea that the therapeutic qualities of a substance can be separated from its physical matter and that these qualities are amplified as the meaning is diluted. The process is thought to imprint the "memory" of the original substance onto the water or alcohol in which it is weakened, with each successive dilution and succussion step increasing this energetic imprint. It's a concept that challenges conventional dose-response relationships found in pharmacology and is often a point of contention for critics.

The implications of potentization extend beyond the mere preparation of remedies. It suggests that healing substances can operate at a level that is subtler than the molecular or chemical; it implies a capacity for water to carry information. This perspective intersects with concepts in quantum physics and the study of water's structure, prompting ongoing debate and research into the nature of water and its potential role in homeopathic potentization.

In practice, the choice of potency is a critical decision for the homeopath and is tailored to each patient. Potencies range from low (such as 1X or 6C, indicating a smaller number of dilutions) to very high (such as 1M or CM, indicating a large number of dilutions). The selection is based on various factors, including the sensitivity of the patient, the nature of the illness, and the duration of the symptoms.

Preparing a homeopathic remedy through potentization also involves an intentionality that practitioners value. Each step is performed with care and precision, as it is believed that the quality of the preparation affects the quality of the healing energy of the remedy. This meticulous process is part of the art and science of homeopathy, reflecting its respect for both the material and non-material aspects of healing.

The Principle of potentiation also indicates the homeopathic view that less is more. By using the smallest dose necessary to stimulate healing, homeopathy seeks to avoid overwhelming the body's vital force and instead gently nudge it towards balance. This minimalistic approach is contrasted with the often high doses of conventional medications that can lead to side effects and toxicity.

Moreover, potentization embodies the homeopathic respect for the complexity and sensitivity of the body. It operates on the understanding that very subtle triggers can activate the body's healing mechanisms and that these mechanisms are capable of profound responses. The tailored potencies speak to this sensitivity, offering a spectrum of stimuli that can be matched to the individual's health and vitality.

The Principle of Potentization also serves to personalize medicine. Since the same substance can be prepared in various potencies, each with its unique profile, it allows for a greater degree of specificity in matching a remedy to a patient's needs. This customization is a testament to the detailed nature of homeopathic practice and its commitment to individualized care.

Within homeopathy, potentization is not merely a means of remedy preparation but also a philosophical stance on the nature of medicine and healing. It posits that energy and information are central to health and that substances have capacities beyond their chemical composition. These principles challenge conventional medical paradigms and invite a broader understanding of what is therapeutically possible.

In summary, The Principle of potentiation is a defining feature of homeopathic medicine, emphasizing energetic dynamics and the belief in the healing power of 'informational' doses. It is a process that underlies the preparation of every homeopathic remedy, contributing to the practice's unique approach to health and its capacity to stimulate the body's self-healing processes with great precision and subtlety.

The Doctrine of Drug Proving: Understanding Remedies through Human Experience

The Doctrine of Drug Proving is a fundamental aspect of homeopathic medicine, whereby the effects of substances are systematically tested on healthy individuals to determine the range of symptoms they produce. These symptoms are meticulously cataloged to create a detailed profile of the remedy's action. This principle ensures that the therapeutic application of homeopathic remedies is grounded in empirical observation and direct human experience rather than theoretical speculation.

Drug proving is based on the premise that understanding a substance's healing capabilities requires knowing the full spectrum of effects it can produce. By observing the symptoms elicited during a proving, homeopaths gain insight into the conditions the substance might treat in a sick person, adhering to the principle of 'like cures like.' This method stands in contrast to conventional drug trials that typically focus on the effects on individuals who are already ill and may not reveal the full potential of the substance.

The Doctrine of Drug Proving reflects a commitment to a democratic and participatory approach to remedy discovery. Provers who volunteer to test the substances come from all walks of life, and their experiences contribute to the collective knowledge of homeopathy. This diversity ensures a comprehensive understanding of remedies, considering variations in symptoms that may arise from individual differences.

During a proving, provers take a homeopathic potency of the substance being tested and record all the changes they experience, whether physical, emotional, or mental. These self-observations require attention and introspection, contributing to the richness of the homeopathic materia medica — the extensive reference to the medicinal properties of substances.

The records from drug provings are compiled and scrutinized by homeopaths to discern patterns and characteristic symptoms that are consistently produced by the substance. These typical symptoms become essential in the homeopathic prescription process as they guide the practitioner in matching a patient's symptoms with the remedy profile.

The Doctrine of Drug Proving is also a testament to the homeopathic respect for the subtlety of human perception and the complexity of human experiences. Unlike conventional trials that may dismiss subjective experiences as irrelevant or anecdotal, homeopathy values these personal reports as essential data for understanding the multi-dimensional impact of remedies.

Drug proving is an ongoing process, reflecting homeopathy's openness to discovering new remedies and expanding its materia medica. As society encounters new substances and our environments change, homeopathy recognizes the need to explore and understand the healing potential of new agents continuously.

The methodology of drug proving also emphasizes safety, as the remedies used are highly diluted, minimizing the risk of adverse effects while eliciting informative symptoms. This cautious approach aligns with the homeopathic principle of primum noncore, "first, not harm," and highlights the discipline's dedication to gentle yet effective therapeutic interventions.

Through drug proving, homeopathy demonstrates an integrative approach to knowledge, combining empirical research with a qualitative understanding of human health. It respects the narratives of individuals as valuable sources of insight, contributing to a medicine that is responsive to the subtleties of human pathology.

In summary, The Doctrine of Drug Proving is a cornerstone of homeopathic practice, offering a systematic and experiential foundation for remedy selection. It provides a framework that respects the nuances of human experiences, emphasizes safety and participation, and underscores the importance of empirical evidence in developing homeopathic therapeutics. This doctrine reinforces homeopathy's dedication to deepening its understanding of healing substances through the direct experiences of those who test them.

Chapter 2: Materia Medica

These are homeopathic remedies derived from various natural sources. The focus is on the mental, emotional, psychological, and physical symptomology associated with the most prescribed homeopathic medicines. By understanding the unique properties and indications of these remedies, practitioners can make well-informed decisions when choosing the most suitable treatment for the patient.

Introduction

Welcome to the profound world of Homeopathic Materia Medica, a pivotal repository of knowledge within homeopathy. This compendium is a guiding light, unveiling the intricate details of medicinal substances derived from nature's vast tapestry. In this comprehensive presentation, we embark on a scholarly exploration of Homeopathic Materia Medica, examining its purpose, structure, historical evolution, interpretation, contemporary perspectives, formulation, principles, detailed list of homeopathic medicines, clinical verification, clinical materia medica, remedy relationships, aggravation and amelioration, modern provings, individualization.

At the heart of homeopathy's therapeutic philosophy lies the principle of 'similia similibus curentur' – like cures. Remedies are chosen based on their ability to induce symptoms in a healthy individual corresponding to those exhibited by a patient. The Materia Medica, a compilation of remedy descriptions and associated symptomatology, is a pivotal guide to this process. It offers an exhaustive catalog of remedy profiles drawn from plant, animal, and mineral sources, detailing their key characteristics, symptoms, and therapeutic indications.

The historical evolution of Homeopathic Materia Medica bears witness to the visionary contributions of pioneers such as Samuel Hahnemann, Constantine Hering, and James Tyler Kent. Hahnemann's foundational work initiated systematic drug proving and laid the groundwork for materia medica compilation. Hering's "law of direction of cure" and emphasis on symptom progression enriched the understanding of healing dynamics. Kent's meticulous approach refined remedy characteristics and constitutional prescribing.

The architecture of Materia Medica entries encompasses botanical or chemical classifications, historical context, provings, and clinical applications. Each remedy is defined by keynote symptoms, modalities (aggravating or ameliorating factors), and accompanying symptoms that provide a holistic view of its effects. Cross-references to related remedies facilitate differentiation and precise prescribing.

Compiling Materia Medica data is a meticulous process drawing from multiple sources – provings, clinical observations, and existing Materia Medica texts. Verification involves confirming symptom authenticity through clinical experience, ensuring the reliability and accuracy of recorded effects. The challenge lies in discerning genuine symptoms from those peripheral or secondary.

Interpreting Materia Medica necessitates a nuanced grasp of symptom hierarchies, modalities, and the totality of a patient's presentation. Repertory symptom indexes aid in narrowing remedy options. Final selection hinges upon the remedy's alignment with the patient's complete symptom profile encompassing physical, mental, and emotional dimensions.

Modern advancements augment the traditional understanding of Materia Medica. Pharmacological studies, molecular research, and clinical trials contribute insights into remedy mechanisms. Moreover, contemporary authors integrate psychology, neurobiology, and psychoneuroimmunology findings, enriching symptomatology interpretation.

Homeopathic Materia Medica is formulated through a meticulous process of drug proving – administering a remedy to healthy individuals and meticulously recording their symptoms. These provings serve as the foundation for remedy profiles, elucidating each substance's effects on various bodily systems. The principles of materia medica involve symptom correspondence, the totality of symptoms, and the law of cure, guiding practitioners toward holistic prescribing.

A comprehensive list of homeopathic medicines encompasses many substances from the natural world, spanning plant, animal, and mineral kingdoms. This compilation details each remedy's symptoms, modalities, and therapeutic applications. From Aconite to Zincum, each remedy's unique profile provides a wealth of information for practitioners to match individualized symptom patterns.

Clinical practitioners validate Materia Medica through real-life case experiences, confirming remedy effectiveness in treating specific conditions. Clinical Materia Medica involves applying remedies in clinical settings, including acute, chronic, and constitutional treatments.

Understanding remedy relationships, such as complementary and similar remedies, enhances prescribing accuracy. Awareness of factors that worsen or alleviate symptoms – aggravation and amelioration – aids in precise remedy selection.

Contemporary approaches employ modern technology and research methodologies for drug proving, refining our understanding of remedies. Individualization, the hallmark of homeopathy, emphasizes tailoring treatment to each patient's unique symptom profile.

The information presented below illustrates Materia Medica's application of inpatient treatment, showcasing the successful alignment of remedies with individual symptoms. In essence, Homeopathic Materia Medica bridges natural substances and human well-being, nurturing holistic health and forming an indispensable cornerstone within the mosaic of homeopathic practice.

What follows is a more comprehensive and extensive description of how homeopathic remedies are created:

Creating Homeopathic Remedies: The Proving Process

Selecting the Substance

The foundation of homeopathic remedies lies in harnessing the potential therapeutic effects of natural substances. These substances encompass a diverse spectrum, ranging from botanical elements to minerals and animal-derived materials. The initial phase involves selecting a sense that possesses relatively uncharted therapeutic attributes. This could encompass a plant species, a mineral variety, an animal-derived compound, or even disease-related components.

Enlisting Healthy Volunteers

Integral to the proving process is recruiting healthy individuals who act as "provers." This cohort is deliberately chosen to be devoid of any pre-existing health issues. This selection criterion ensures that existing health conditions do not confound the effects of the substance under investigation. The provers serve as a controlled baseline for observing the substance's impact.

Administration of Prepared Substance

The selected substance is subjected to a specialized preparation. This involves a sequence of dilutions and potentizations. This procedure renders the importance safe yet highly potent. Dilution is coupled with vigorous shaking, a process known as "succussion," which imparts distinctive properties to homeopathic remedies.

Cataloging Changes and Reactions

The provers embark on a regimen of the prepared remedy, meticulously documenting any physiological, psychological, or emotional changes. These observations encompass alterations in sleep patterns, shifts in mood, variations in energy levels, and any other nuanced experiences. The objective is to capture a comprehensive spectrum of reactions.

Diverse Individual Responses

A fascinating facet of the proving process is the diversity of responses exhibited by each prover. While commonalities might emerge, the individualized nature of reactions underscores the substance's multifaceted interaction with the human organism.

Compilation and Analysis of Data

At the culmination of the proving period, the extensive journals maintained by the provers are collated. These journals serve as a repository of valuable data, capturing the intricacies of individual experiences. The data thus amassed becomes the foundation for meticulous analysis.

Discerning Patterns and Effects

Practitioners engage in a systematic analysis of the aggregated data. The aim is to discern patterns – recurring symptoms and responses shared across different provers. These patterns form the basis for comprehending the substance's potential impact on physiological, psychological, and emotional domains.

Development of the Homeopathic Remedy

Equipped with a nuanced understanding of the substance's effects, developing a homeopathic remedy ensues. This remedy encapsulates the essence of the importance, achieved through extensive dilution and potentization. The remedy's preparation embodies the substance's therapeutic spirit.

Customized Healing

In clinical application, a homeopathic practitioner tailors treatment to the individual's symptoms, constitution, and health profile. When a patient's symptoms align with those exhibited by the provers during the proving, the corresponding homeopathic remedy is administered. This remedy triggers the body's intrinsic healing response, fostering a personalized path to recovery.

Essentially, the proving process is a scientific exploration of nature's potential healing capabilities. It amalgamates the intricacies of human physiology with the nuanced interactions between substances and the body's innate healing mechanisms. Homeopathic remedies, thus derived, exemplify the fusion of empirical observation and therapeutic innovation.

A list of the most prescribed homeopathic remedies:

Medical Disclaimer: Homeopathic Remedies and Alternative Medicine

This content, including all discussions, suggestions, and references to homeopathic remedies and alternative medicine, is provided strictly for entertainment and informational purposes only. It is not intended as medical advice, nor should it be used as a substitute for consultations with qualified healthcare professionals familiar with your medical needs.

If you are considering combining homeopathic remedies with conventional medical treatments, it is crucial to consult a licensed healthcare professional. Only a qualified healthcare provider can advise on what is safe and effective for your unique health needs and diagnose and treat medical conditions.

Any decisions regarding your health or medical treatments should be made in partnership with a licensed healthcare professional. The creators and distributors of this content disclaim any liability for any harm or adverse effects resulting from using or applying the information provided here. Viewer discretion is advised, and viewers are encouraged to consult a medical professional before adopting alternative health practices.

Remember: This content is for entertainment and should not be taken as medical advice.

Materia, Medica

The following are some of the more widely prescribed homeopathic remedies.

Aconite (Aconitum Napellus)

• Mental: Aconite is significant for its profound impact on the mental state, often in cases of acute fear and anxiety. This remedy is chosen for sudden and intense conditions, especially following shock or fright. Patients may experience an extreme sense of restlessness and an acute fear of death, with a preoccupation with mortality. This remedy suits conditions arising from emotional and physical stressors, such as exposure to cold or traumatic events.

• Emotional: Aconite affects individuals who experience intense fear and anxiety with any ailment. There's a sense of foreboding about the future. The emotional state may include uncontrolled stress leading to physical symptoms. Aconite is also helpful for symptoms arising from exposure to cold and dry weather, causing emotional distress.

• Psychological: Psychologically, Aconite affects patients with heightened tension from both emotional and physical stressors. It's the first choice in acute diseases and inflammatory conditions before pathological changes occur. The psychological profile includes a hyper-acute state of mind with exaggerated responses.

• Physical: Aconite addresses acute conditions with symptoms like tingling, coldness, numbness, and sudden weakness. It's effective for influenza and infections involving serous membranes and muscular tissues. It's often indicated in the early stages of fever, inflammation, and symptoms from cold drafts or temperature changes.

Acid Phos (Phosphoricum Acidum)

• Mental: Acid Phos profoundly affects mental faculties, often leading to impaired memory and difficulty in comprehension. It is particularly effective in treating conditions following mental shock or grief, manifesting as an inability to collect thoughts or find the right words. This remedy is suited for individuals who experience a significant decline in cognitive function after emotional trauma.

• Emotional: Emotionally, Acid Phos is indicated for deep-rooted sadness and depression, often arising from emotional trauma like grief or heartbreak. Patients may exhibit an aversion to mental work and demonstrate a general emotional indifference, reflecting an overall disengagement from life activities.

• Psychological: Psychologically, Acid Phos addresses the impact of intense emotions such as grief, disappointment, or heartache. This remedy is known for its effectiveness in treating the psychological aftermath of emotional suffering, where the individual experiences a loss of motivation or drive, often leading to a significant reduction in life's activities.

• Physical: On the physical level, Acid Phos is commonly used for conditions of debility and exhaustion that follow emotional trauma. It is particularly effective in cases where physical and mental fatigue are exacerbated by a period of emotional distress, grief, or disappointment. This remedy helps in restoring energy levels and improving overall physical vitality.

Allium Cepa

• Mental: Allium Cepa has a significant impact on mental processes, often causing confusion and difficulty concentrating. It is particularly effective in conditions with reduced cognitive abilities, such as processing thoughts or finding the right words, especially following exposure to allergens or during colds. This remedy addresses the mental fog and disorientation commonly experienced with upper respiratory ailments.

• Emotional: Emotionally, Allium Cepa benefits individuals who experience profound sadness, despair, and discontent, often as a response to physical discomfort. It's helpful in cases where emotional turmoil is linked with the physical symptoms of respiratory issues. This remedy aids in stabilizing the emotional responses triggered by the discomfort of colds or allergies.

• Psychological: Psychologically, Allium Cepa helps in cases where there is a compounding of mental depression due to persistent physical symptoms. It is effective in alleviating the psychological distress associated with chronic or acute respiratory ailments, improving the overall mental state of individuals suffering from these conditions.

• Physical: Physically, Allium Cepa is renowned for its efficacy in treating symptoms of the common cold or hay fever, like watery eyes and a runny nose, especially when aggravated in warm environments and alleviated in open air. It also addresses the sharp, biting sensations in the eyes and nose, providing relief from these common colds or allergic reactions.

Antimonium Crudum (Antim Crud)

• Mental: Antimonium Crudum significantly impacts mental states, particularly in cases of irritability, moodiness, and melancholy. This remedy is often chosen for individuals generally dissatisfied with life, especially when linked to digestive disturbances. It addresses the mental fog and disorientation that can accompany gastrointestinal distress.

• Emotional: Emotionally, Antim Crud is effective for treating heightened emotional sensitivity, often linked to physical discomfort or dietary indiscretions. It's used for patients experiencing mood swings or who become easily upset, particularly after overindulgence in food or with specific nutritional sensitivities.

• Psychological: Psychologically, this remedy assists in cases where emotional disturbances are closely tied to physical ailments, particularly gastrointestinal. It aids in moderating psychological responses associated with physical discomfort, bringing about emotional stability in the context of physical health issues.

• Physical: Physically, Antimonium Crudum is used for conditions like indigestion, characterized by symptoms like nausea or a coated tongue. It's also beneficial in treating skin conditions such as eczema or sensitive calluses, offering relief from the discomfort associated with these issues.

Antimonium Tartaricum (Antim Tart)

• Mental: Antimonium Tartaricum impacts the mental state, particularly noted for inducing confusion and drowsiness. It's chosen for individuals with a passive mental state, often seen in conjunction with respiratory conditions. This remedy addresses mental sluggishness and a lack of alertness, especially in elderly patients or during respiratory illnesses.

• Emotional: Emotionally, Antim Tart treats emotional irritation and distress linked with physical respiratory symptoms. It's suitable for patients who exhibit irritability or emotional sensitivity, particularly in response to respiratory discomfort or fatigue.

• Psychological: Psychologically, Antim Tart assists in cases where mental and emotional disturbances correlate with physical respiratory conditions. It helps in stabilizing the psychological responses arising from respiratory discomfort, illness, or the feeling of being overwhelmed by physical symptoms.

• Physical: On the physical front, Antimonium Tartaricum is renowned for its effectiveness in respiratory conditions with congestive symptoms, like heavy mucus in the chest. It's beneficial in bronchitis, respiratory infections with mucus production, and when there is difficulty in expectorating mucus.

Apis Mellifica (Apis Mell.)

• Mental: Apis Mellifica significantly affects mental conditions, often leading to agitation and restlessness. It's particularly effective for individuals who exhibit a lack of focus and a sense of mental overwhelm, especially in acute conditions. This remedy is suitable for those experiencing rapid shifts in mental states and difficulty in maintaining mental composure.

• Emotional: Emotionally, Apis Mell. Treats states of emotional volatility linked to physical symptoms like swelling or pain. It benefits patients with sudden emotional outbursts or heightened sensitivity in response to physical discomfort, particularly in inflammatory conditions.

• Psychological: Psychologically, Apis Mell. Assists in situations with a correlation between mental and emotional disturbances and physical conditions. It helps moderate psychological responses associated with physical discomfort, especially inflammation or allergic reactions.

• Physical: Physically, Apis Mellifica is renowned for treating swelling, redness, and stinging pain, similar to bee stings. It's beneficial in acute inflammatory conditions, allergic reactions, and fluid retention cases, offering relief from these specific physical symptoms.

Arnica

• Mental: Arnica significantly impacts the mental state, particularly in cases of shock or trauma. It is commonly indicated for individuals who experience mental disorientation or confusion after an injury or traumatic event. This remedy benefits those feeling mentally dizzy and unable to process events usually.

• Emotional: Emotionally, Arnica is effective in treating emotional distress associated with physical injuries or trauma. Patients may exhibit emotional detachment or denial about their condition, often insisting they are fine despite clear signs of damage or pain.

• Psychological: Psychologically, Arnica assists in stabilizing the mental and emotional responses to physical trauma. It is helpful in conditions where psychological disturbances result from injuries, surgeries, or physical shocks, aiding in the emotional processing of traumatic experiences.

• Physical: Physically, Arnica is renowned for its effectiveness in bruising, swelling, and pain, particularly related to trauma or soft tissue injury. It is also widely used post-surgery to reduce inflammation and accelerate the healing process, aiding in recovery from physical trauma.

Argentum Nitricum

• Mental: Argentum Nitricum is extensively used for managing anxiety, particularly anxiety linked with future events or performances. This remedy is ideal for individuals experiencing nervous anticipation, often manifesting in hurried and impulsive behaviors. It also addresses mental states with a sense of hurriedness and a lack of control over thoughts.

• Emotional: It significantly addresses intense nervousness and emotional impulsiveness. People who benefit from this remedy often exhibit heightened emotional responses to stress and may experience sudden bouts of anxiety or fear without a clear cause.

• Psychological: This remedy is effective for various irrational fears and phobias, such as fear of flying, claustrophobia, or fear of failure. It helps reduce the psychological impact of these fears, assisting individuals in coping with situations that trigger their anxieties.

• Physical: Argentum Nitricum is widely used for digestive disturbances linked to nervousness, such as gas, bloating, and diarrhea, and is particularly effective when these symptoms worsen with sugar. It also addresses physical symptoms that manifest under stress, such as trembling or palpitations.

Belladonna
• Mental: Belladonna is widely used for acute mental conditions characterized by fever, delirium, and hallucinations. It's effective for intense agitation, confusion, and cases where there's a sudden onset of cognitive symptoms. This remedy is also used in situations of manic behavior or when there's an intense reaction to sensory stimuli.
• Emotional: Emotionally, Belladonna addresses extreme emotional responses such as fright, rage, or intense fear. It's beneficial in cases where emotional symptoms appear suddenly and with great intensity, often accompanying physical symptoms.
• Psychological: Psychologically, Belladonna is critical in managing acute psychological disturbances like delusions, vivid hallucinations, and extreme fearfulness. This remedy is particularly indicated in sensitive situations with rapid shifts in psychological states, often accompanying high fever or physical pain.
• Physical: Belladonna is known for treating symptoms of high fever, redness, throbbing pain, inflammation, and acute infections. It's typically used in conditions like sudden fever spikes, earaches, sore throats, pounding headaches, and any inflammatory disorder with a rapid onset.

Bellis Perennis
• Mental: Bellis Perennis addresses profound mental lethargy and fatigue, mainly resulting from physical overexertion. It is beneficial for those who feel mentally drained, unable to

concentrate, or mentally foggy after strenuous physical activities or injuries.

• Emotional: On an emotional level, this remedy offers relief from the low mood or emotional fatigue that frequently follows extensive physical work or trauma. It's helpful for emotional exhaustion directly tied to physical labor or injuries.

• Psychological: Psychologically, Bellis Perennis assists in cases of mental overwhelm or exhaustion following physically demanding tasks or injuries. It supports the recovery of mental energy and resilience, aiding those who have undergone physically taxing situations.

• Physical: For physical ailments, Bellis Perennis excels in treating injuries to deeper tissues, such as significant bruises, sprains, and post-surgical recovery. It's also effective in alleviating general body soreness, aches, and fatigue from extensive physical exertion, making it a vital remedy for recovery from physically demanding activities or deep bodily traumas.

Berberis Vulgaris

• Mental: Berberis Vulgaris is used for conditions where mental fatigue or lethargy is prominent, often in connection with kidney or bladder issues. It's helpful for those experiencing a lack of mental clarity or sluggish cognitive functioning, which may be related to underlying physical conditions.

• Emotional: This remedy is effective for emotional irritability and frustration, particularly when these emotions are tied to physical discomfort like urinary problems. It helps in managing mood swings and emotional distress related to physical ailments.

• Psychological: Psychologically, Berberis Vulgaris can aid individuals feeling mentally overwhelmed or drained, often due to chronic physical conditions like urinary tract issues or renal problems. It supports mental well-being in the context of ongoing physical health issues.

• Physical: Known for its efficacy in treating kidney and bladder conditions, including kidney stones and urinary tract infections, Berberis Vulgaris also addresses the pain and discomfort associated with these conditions. It's beneficial for alleviating symptoms like sharp, radiating pains and is often used in managing chronic urinary conditions.

Bryonia

• Mental: Bryonia is typically chosen for individuals who experience significant irritability and a strong preference for solitude when unwell. It's particularly effective for those who become easily frustrated or agitated due to physical discomfort or illness.

• Emotional: Emotionally, this remedy is suited for managing states with a heightened need for stability and an aversion to change, which often becomes more pronounced during illness. It aids in stabilizing emotions during periods of physical health challenges.

• Psychological: Psychologically, Bryonia assists individuals who are overwhelmed or anxious about their health, especially in chronic illnesses. It helps in reducing the stress and anxiety that often accompany prolonged physical conditions.

• Physical: Known for its efficacy in treating conditions like dry coughs, joint pains, and digestive problems, Bryonia is especially valuable when symptoms intensify with movement. It's also practical for headaches, constipation, and other issues related to dehydration or dryness.

Cactus

• Mental: Cactus is particularly effective for mental states marked by a sensation of constriction or oppression. It's used in cases where emotional stress manifests in a feeling of mental tightness or being trapped.

• Emotional: Emotionally, this remedy is suited for feelings of heaviness or emotional suffocation, often linked with heart conditions or intense emotional distress. It helps individuals who feel emotionally constricted or burdened.

• Psychological: Psychologically, Cactus benefits those who experience overwhelming feelings or a sense of being trapped in their emotional state. It helps alleviate the psychological impact of emotional and physical stress.

• Physical: Known for treating heart-related symptoms like palpitations, chest pain, or sensations of tightness, Cactus is also beneficial in conditions with a physical sense of constriction, whether in the chest or other areas.

Calcarea Carb

• Mental: Calcarea Carb is highly effective for mental conditions marked by anxiety and worry, particularly about health, security, and routine life tasks. It's often chosen for individuals who feel overwhelmed by responsibilities and fear unforeseen changes. This remedy aids those who are generally cautious yet struggle with internal anxieties about their capabilities and future.

• Emotional: Emotionally, this remedy is tailored for those facing fears of instability and failure and is familiar to individuals who frequently worry about their future and security. Calcarea Carb helps alleviate these deep-seated emotional concerns, providing stability and groundedness.

• Psychological: Psychologically, Calcarea Carb assists individuals overwhelmed by life's demands. It's beneficial for those who experience stress from personal and professional responsibilities, offering support in maintaining mental and emotional equilibrium in the face of challenges.

• Physical: On the physical front, Calcarea Carb is renowned for addressing metabolic and developmental issues, such as bone and teeth problems, and is also used for fatigue, weakness, and susceptibility to cold. It's instrumental in managing physical symptoms that manifest due to metabolic imbalances.

Calcarea Fluor

• Mental: Calcarea Fluor is adept at addressing mental states marked by rigidity and a deep-seated fear of financial loss or instability. It's beneficial for those who feel mentally constricted by worries related to material security, manifesting as an inability to adapt to changing circumstances or new ideas.

• Emotional: Emotionally, this remedy is tailored for those burdened by the stress of responsibilities, especially where these concerns are linked to maintaining stability and security. It supports individuals overwhelmed by the emotional weight of financial and duty-related worries.

• Psychological: Psychologically, Calcarea Fluor assists individuals who struggle with adapting to change and facing significant stress due to a rigid or inflexible mindset. It helps alleviate the discomfort associated with an unwillingness or inability to embrace new perspectives or challenges.

• Physical: On the physical front, Calcarea Fluor is well-regarded for its efficacy in treating bone and joint issues, such as joint pains, bone spurs, and dental health concerns like tooth decay. It plays a significant role in dental health, particularly in strengthening tooth enamel and combating dental decay.

Calcarea Phos

• Mental: Calcarea Phos is particularly effective for mental fatigue and dissatisfaction or restlessness common in growing children and adolescents. It helps address issues like difficulty concentrating, feeling mentally overwhelmed due to physical changes, and general unease often accompanying developmental stages.

• Emotional: This remedy is tailored for emotional challenges during growth phases, such as irritability, mood swings, and discontent commonly observed during growth spurts in children and teenagers. It assists in stabilizing emotional responses associated with the pressures of physical and social changes.

• Psychological: Psychologically, Calcarea Phos benefits those overwhelmed by the rapid changes associated with growth and development. It's beneficial for easing the stress and anxiety accompanying these periods, offering support for psychological well-being during significant developmental changes.

• Physical: Known for its effectiveness in bone and teeth health, mainly during rapid growth, Calcarea Phos is extensively used for healing fractures, aiding recovery, and addressing conditions like teething pains or bone weakness. It plays a critical role in supporting the physical development of bones and teeth in children and adolescents.

Calcarea Sulph

• Mental: Calcarea Sulph is primarily used for mental conditions such as dullness and sluggishness, typically seen after prolonged illness or chronic infections. It addresses deep-seated mental fatigue and a lack of concentration, often a residual effect of lengthy health struggles.

• Emotional: This remedy assists in emotional regulation, particularly irritability and discontent, familiar during convalescence or with chronic health issues. It aids in stabilizing emotional upheaval during recovery phases, helping individuals manage feelings of frustration and dissatisfaction linked to their health state.

• Psychological: Psychologically, Calcarea Sulph supports those burdened by long-term health challenges. It is instrumental in coping with the mental strain and emotional toll associated with extended recovery periods, helping individuals navigate the psychological impact of their health journey.

• Physical: Renowned for its efficacy in skin conditions such as acne, abscesses, and slow-healing wounds, Calcarea Sulph is also crucial in treating diseases with pus formation or discharge. Its role in supporting the body's natural healing processes, especially in skin-related conditions, is significant, aiding overall recovery.

Calendula

• Mental: Calendula offers nuanced mental benefits, notably in soothing the mental disturbances that accompany physical injuries. It provides a calming influence on the mind, particularly beneficial during recovery from physical trauma, reducing the cognitive burden and enhancing focus on healing.

• Emotional: Emotionally, Calendula is invaluable for alleviating distress related to skin injuries, surgical recovery, and other physical traumas. It helps stabilize emotional fluctuations during recovery, fostering a sense of emotional resilience and well-being.

• Psychological: In terms of psychological health, Calendula is effective in mitigating the stress and trauma associated with physical injuries. It aids individuals in coping with the psychological aftermath of physical trauma, supporting a healthier recovery process.

• Physical: The physical benefits of Calendula are extensive, encompassing the healing of various types of skin wounds, burns, and more profound tissue damage. Its antiseptic and healing properties make it an essential component in natural wound care, promoting efficient and healthy skin recovery.

Cantharis

• Mental: Cantharis is particularly effective for mental irritation and restlessness, often seen in individuals with urinary tract conditions. It addresses a heightened mental unease, agitation, and irritability commonly associated with intense physical discomfort.

• Emotional: Emotionally, this remedy is crucial for managing volatility and heightened sensitivity. It's beneficial for individuals who react emotionally to physical discomfort or irritation, helping to stabilize mood swings and emotional responses linked to physical ailments.

• Psychological: Psychologically, Cantharis aids those experiencing stress or agitation from acute physical conditions. It offers relief to individuals struggling with the psychological impact of painful and uncomfortable physical symptoms.

• Physical: Cantharis is renowned for treating conditions like urinary tract infections, burns, and scalds. It is effective in alleviating intense pain, burning sensations, and discomfort during urination, making it an essential remedy in cases of severe physical irritation.

Carbo Veg

• Mental: Carbo Veg addresses profound mental fatigue and a sense of deep lethargy, often a result of illness, overexertion, or exhaustion. This remedy is particularly suited for those experiencing a significant reduction in mental energy and clarity, impacting their ability to engage in daily tasks.

• Emotional: On an emotional level, Carbo Veg benefits individuals who experience emotional numbness or indifference, a common aftermath of prolonged illness or fatigue. It aids in reinvigorating emotional responsiveness and alleviating feelings of emotional detachment.

• Psychological: Psychologically, this remedy relieves individuals overwhelmed by a lack of vitality. It helps restore psychological energy and vigor, which is especially useful for those recovering from physical or emotional depletion.

• Physical: Known for its efficacy in digestive ailments and respiratory conditions, Carbo Veg is particularly effective in alleviating symptoms like bloating, gas, and indigestion. It's also valuable in managing general physical weakness, aiding the body's recovery and energy restoration.

Caulophyllum

• Mental: While Caulophyllum is not primarily focused on mental symptoms, it can be supportive in alleviating mental stress, particularly when related to menstrual issues or the process of childbirth. It helps manage the mental aspects of gynecological health, such as stress or worry.

• Emotional: Emotionally, this remedy helps address the fluctuations often associated with menstrual cycles or childbirth. It assists in stabilizing emotional responses and helps manage mood swings related to hormonal changes.

• Psychological: Psychologically, Caulophyllum aids in coping with stress and anxiety, especially those linked to gynecological health or childbirth. It offers support to women dealing with the psychological impact of menstrual disorders or labor difficulties.

• Physical: Caulophyllum is renowned for treating menstrual disorders, difficulties during labor, and joint pains, particularly in the small joints. It's effective in easing menstrual cramps irregular cycles and assisting with childbirth-related issues.

Chamomilla

• Mental: Chamomilla is beneficial for managing irritability and restlessness, especially in children. It addresses conditions of hypersensitivity to pain, where even minor discomfort can lead to significant mental agitation. This remedy is often chosen for its ability to calm the mind in heightened sensitivity.

• Emotional: Emotionally, Chamomilla treats sudden emotional outbursts such as anger or irritability. These responses are often observed in cases of pain or discomfort, making Chamomilla ideal for soothing emotional turmoil in such scenarios.

• Psychological: Psychologically, this remedy aids in managing the stress and frustration accompanying pain or illness. It's constructive for children who may find it challenging to cope with the psychological aspects of physical discomfort.

• Physical: Known for its efficacy in treating teething pain in infants, Chamomilla is also widely used for menstrual cramps, earaches, and other conditions characterized by intense pain. It is helpful when the pain response seems disproportionate to the cause.

China Officinalis

• Mental: China Officinalis is extensively used for profound mental fatigue and debility, especially after illness, significant blood loss, or profound exhaustion. It addresses conditions where mental capacity is severely diminished due to physical strain or depletion, helping to restore mental alertness and clarity.

• Emotional: This remedy is particularly effective in managing heightened emotional sensitivity and irritability in those weakened by illness or fluid loss. It aids in stabilizing emotional fluctuations and relieves the irritability often associated with physical weakening.

• Psychological: Psychologically, China Officinalis supports individuals feeling profoundly drained or overwhelmed due to extensive physical debilitation. It assists in rejuvenating psychological vigor and aids in coping with the mental aspects of recovery from illness or fluid loss.

• Physical: Recognized for treating conditions resulting from significant fluid loss, such as bleeding, severe diarrhea, or profuse sweating, China Officinalis is also known for its therapeutic effects in cases of physical weakness and exhaustion. It is commonly used to replenish the body's strength after episodes of substantial fluid depletion or in the aftermath of chronic illnesses.

Cimicifuga

• Mental: Cimicifuga is extensively used for more profound mental symptoms such as severe depression and heightened anxiety, mainly related to hormonal fluctuations during menstrual cycles or menopause. It's effective in addressing intense feelings of despair and fluctuating anxiety levels that correlate with hormonal changes.

• Emotional: This remedy excels in managing significant emotional upheavals, including pronounced mood swings and irritability often linked to menstrual and menopausal phases. It offers stability and relief from emotional turbulence during these hormonal transitions.

• Psychological: Psychologically, Cimicifuga is invaluable for easing stress or tension stemming from gynecological issues. It aids in coping with the psychological challenges and stressors associated with menstrual discomfort and menopausal changes.

• Physical: Cimicifuga's role in women's health extends to effectively treating severe menstrual cramps, intense premenstrual syndrome, and challenging menopausal symptoms, including substantial joint and muscle pain. Its importance in alleviating physical discomfort associated with hormonal shifts is significant.

Cocculus Indicus

- Mental: Cocculus Indicus is highly effective for more profound mental symptoms such as severe dizziness, marked confusion, and significant cognitive disturbances often linked to motion sickness or severe sleep deprivation. It addresses intense mental disorientation and the inability to focus or think clearly under these conditions.

- Emotional: Emotionally, this remedy is critical for addressing deep-seated anxiety and feelings of weakness, particularly during extended periods of physical or mental stress. It aids in balancing emotional responses to extreme fatigue or stress.

- Psychological: Psychologically, Cocculus Indicus is invaluable for those overwhelmed by intense fatigue or stress, helping to manage the psychological impact of these conditions. It provides support in coping with mental and emotional exhaustion.

- Physical: Cocculus Indicus is renowned for its effectiveness in addressing severe symptoms of motion sickness, vertigo, and intense nausea. It is also extensively used for treating significant muscle weakness and exhaustion. The remedy is beneficial for counteracting physical symptoms arising from stress, travel, or lack of rest.

Colocynthis

- Mental: Colocynthis deeply addresses mental anguish and heightened irritability, mainly stemming from severe abdominal pain or complex digestive issues. It focuses on alleviating the mental distress that often accompanies intense physical discomfort, offering relief from the mental turmoil caused by chronic or acute pain.

- Emotional: This remedy is crucial for managing profound emotional distress, frequently a response to acute physical pain. It assists in stabilizing emotional upheavals and mitigating the solid emotional reactions often linked to physical suffering.

- Psychological: Colocynthis is beneficial for individuals experiencing substantial psychological stress or frustration due to intense physical discomfort. It helps in relieving the psychological impacts associated with persistent or severe pain.
- Physical: Colocynthis is renowned for treating acute abdominal cramps, neuralgia, and sciatica. It is adept at alleviating intense shooting pains and severe gastrointestinal discomfort, making it an essential remedy for managing debilitating physical pain.

Conium Maculatum
- Mental: Conium Maculatum deeply addresses more complex mental symptoms such as advanced confusion, significant cognitive slowing, and memory decline, typically seen in older adults. It's specifically tailored to mitigate the effects of mental deterioration and to support cognitive function in older adults.
- Emotional: Emotionally, this remedy is pivotal in managing profound states of depression and intense fears, including the fear of solitude and isolation that often affects older individuals. It provides substantial relief from these emotional challenges that accompany aging.
- Psychological: On a psychological level, Conium Maculatum is beneficial for those grappling with feelings of stagnation or fear of aging and physical decline. It assists in addressing the psychological implications of aging and helping older individuals cope with the mental and emotional aspects of this life stage.
- Physical: Conium Maculatum's effectiveness extends to treating various age-related physical conditions. It's beneficial for glandular issues, pronounced cases of vertigo, and significant weakness. This remedy is crucial in managing and alleviating the physical ailments associated with aging.

Cuprum Metallicum

• Mental: Cuprum Metallicum is extensively used to address severe mental symptoms like deep nervousness, intense agitation, and heightened anxiety, particularly related to neuromuscular disorders and muscle spasms. It focuses on alleviating the profound mental discomfort and distress that often accompany these physical issues.

• Emotional: This remedy effectively manages profound emotional states, such as intense fear or anxiety, especially those connected to physical conditions like convulsive episodes or severe muscle cramps. It assists in stabilizing and moderating these strong emotional reactions to physical ailments.

• Psychological: Psychologically, Cuprum Metallicum is instrumental for those grappling with significant stress or anxiety resulting from ongoing muscular or nervous system conditions. It supports individuals in coping with the psychological effects and challenges of these chronic health problems.

• Physical: Recognized for treating extreme muscle spasms, intense cramps, and various convulsive disorders, Cuprum Metallicum is also highly effective in managing respiratory conditions like asthma with spasmodic symptoms. It provides substantial relief from the physical manifestations of these conditions.

Digitalis

• Mental: Digitalis is extensively used for managing profound anxiety and deep-rooted fears, especially those related to the fear of death and severe cardiac concerns. It effectively addresses the intense stress and worry often linked to heart disorders, providing relief in situations where cardiac health is a significant concern.

• Emotional: On an emotional level, this remedy significantly aids in dealing with severe depression and melancholy, particularly when these emotional states are connected to heart diseases. It helps alleviate the emotional distress associated with chronic cardiac conditions.

• Psychological: Psychologically, Digitalis is invaluable for individuals facing substantial stress and anxiety due to heart-related issues. It assists in managing the psychological impact of cardiac health concerns, offering support and relief.

• Physical: Digitalis is recognized for its effectiveness in a wide range of heart conditions, including palpitations, arrhythmias, and heart failure, as well as in cases with slow pulse rates. Its role in the comprehensive management of various cardiac conditions is critical.

Eupatorium Perfoliatum

• Mental: While not primarily used for mental conditions, Eupatorium Perfoliatum can alleviate mental discomfort that often accompanies severe body aches or flu-like symptoms, helping to reduce the overall sense of malaise and mental distress associated with physical illness.

• Emotional: This remedy effectively addresses the emotional distress that often occurs with intense physical discomfort, such as high fever or severe body aches. It aids in managing the emotional turmoil related to acute physical health conditions.

• Psychological: Psychologically, Eupatorium Perfoliatum assists in alleviating stress and concern related to severe flu symptoms or bodily pain, offering support in coping with the psychological aspects of illness.

• Physical: Known for its efficacy in treating flu symptoms, Eupatorium Perfoliatum is particularly effective against high fever, severe body aches, and chills, making it a go-to remedy for flu-like conditions.

Ferrum phosphoricum

- Mental: While not primarily used for mental conditions, Ferrum Phosphoricum may help alleviate mental fatigue accompanying physical weakness or the onset of fever. It is suited for those experiencing a lack of mental vigor due to mild physical ailments.

- Emotional: Emotionally, this remedy helps address fatigue or a general lack of energy, mainly linked to conditions like anemia or the early stages of fever. It helps in managing emotional weariness associated with physical debilitation.

- Psychological: Psychologically, Ferrum Phosphoricum can aid individuals who are feeling generally unwell or are in the initial stages of an illness. It supports coping with the psychological aspects of feeling physically under the weather.

- Physical: It is most known for its effectiveness in the early stages of fever, inflammation, and respiratory issues. Ferrum phosphoricum is also commonly used in cases of anemia and physical weakness, helping to address these conditions by enhancing the body's strength and vitality.

Gelsemium

- Mental: Gelsemium is particularly effective for mental symptoms like dizziness, mental dullness, and lethargy, often seen in cases of anxiety or anticipation. It's used when there's a mental fog or sluggishness due to nervousness about upcoming events.

- Emotional: This remedy is beneficial in addressing emotional states of deep apprehension or fear, especially those related to future events or stress. It helps in calming and stabilizing the emotional responses associated with anxiety.

• Psychological: Psychologically, Gelsemium aids in managing overwhelming anxiety or the sensation of being paralyzed by fear, particularly concerning future events. It supports individuals coping with the psychological aspects of apprehension and stress.

• Physical: Known for treating flu-like symptoms characterized by fatigue, heaviness, and muscle weakness, Gelsemium is also effective for headaches and nervous disorders. It addresses the physical manifestations of anxiety and stress.

Hepar Sulph

• Mental: Hepar Sulph is highly effective for addressing pronounced irritability and acute sensitivity, especially in situations involving overreaction to minor annoyances or stimuli. It targets the heightened mental responses to minor irritants.

• Emotional: Emotionally, this remedy is crucial for managing significant volatility and a tendency toward rapid anger or irritability, even in response to seemingly inconsequential issues. It assists in moderating these intense emotional reactions.

• Psychological: Psychologically, heparsulph supports individuals who quickly become overwhelmed or angered by minor disturbances, aiding in the management of these disproportionate psychological reactions.

• Physical: Recognized for its effectiveness in treating skin conditions like abscesses and boils, Hepar Sulph is also used for respiratory diseases with a heightened sensitivity to cold and proneness to infection.

Hypericum Perforatum

• Mental: Hypericum is extensively utilized for its efficacy in mitigating mental distress often linked to nerve pain. It's instrumental in addressing not just the physical aspects of nerve-related discomfort but also the consequential mental agitation and cognitive disturbances that can arise from such pain.

• Emotional: Emotionally, Hypericum plays a crucial role in managing the spectrum of emotional responses triggered by nerve pain, especially of a shooting or stabbing nature. It provides significant emotional relief and stabilization in response to the intense discomfort associated with nerve damage or irritation.

• Psychological: On a psychological level, Hypericum is vital for assisting individuals in coping with the considerable stress and psychological ramifications of nerve pain or injuries. It supports the mental health aspects of dealing with nerve-related conditions, helping to alleviate the psychological burden that often accompanies such injuries.

• Physical: Hypericum's physical applications are notably diverse, especially in treating injuries to nerve-rich areas like fingers, toes, and the spinal region. It's particularly efficacious for conditions involving sharp shooting pains and nerve injuries, making it an indispensable remedy in the realm of nerve-related trauma and neuropathic pain.

Ignatia Amara

• Mental: Ignatia Amara is widely used for treating mental symptoms such as acute emotional distress, particularly related to grief or emotional shock. It addresses symptoms like mood swings and hypersensitivity to emotional stimuli.

• Emotional: This remedy is particularly effective in managing deep emotional reactions, including acute grief, anxiety, or sadness, often following emotional trauma or loss.

• Psychological: Psychologically, Ignatia Amara aids in coping with the complex psychological effects of emotional upheaval, offering relief from the stress and mental strain caused by intense emotional experiences.

• Physical: Physically, Ignatia Amara is known to help with symptoms like nervous headaches, spasms, and other stress-related physical manifestations.

Kali Bichromicum

• Mental: While Kali Bichromicum's primary effects are not on mental health, it can be instrumental in alleviating mental fog or sluggish cognitive function often associated with sinus issues or head colds. It addresses the cognitive dullness patients with chronic sinusitis or upper respiratory conditions might experience.

• Emotional: Emotionally, this remedy manages symptoms such as irritability or a low mood that may accompany chronic respiratory conditions like sinusitis. It can help stabilize mood disturbances related to ongoing respiratory issues.

• Psychological: Psychologically, Kali Bichromicum aids individuals who feel mentally burdened or overwhelmed due to persistent respiratory issues. It supports managing the psychological strain often accompanying chronic sinus and respiratory conditions.

• Physical: Known for its effectiveness in treating conditions with thick, stringy mucus discharges, Kali Bichromicum is particularly beneficial in sinusitis and stubborn respiratory infections. It is specifically indicated for sinus and throat issues where the mucus is viscous and tenacious.

Kali Bichromicum is notable for its role in managing respiratory conditions, particularly those characterized by specific mucus discharges, and its implications for mental, emotional, and psychological health.

Lachesis

• Mental: Lachesis is frequently utilized for addressing complex mental symptoms like intense jealousy, deep-rooted suspicion, and excessive talkativeness, often linked to hormonal imbalances or circulatory issues. It's particularly effective when these mental states are pronounced and impact daily functioning.

• Emotional: Emotionally, this remedy is adept at managing volatile emotional states, including significant irritability and mood fluctuations, commonly observed in conditions like menopausal or premenstrual syndromes. It helps in stabilizing these emotional swings.

• Psychological: Psychologically, Lachesis aids in managing feelings of oppression, paranoia, or extreme emotional distress, especially concerning hormonal or circulatory conditions. It offers support in coping with the psychological effects of these health issues.

• Physical: Known for treating conditions related to poor circulation and various inflammatory issues, Lachesis is also highly effective in managing menopausal symptoms. It addresses a range of physical symptoms associated with hormonal and circulatory imbalances.

Lachesis is notable for its wide-ranging effects in conditions involving hormonal changes and circulatory issues, with significant implications for mental, emotional, psychological, and physical health.

Ledum Palustre

• Mental: While not primarily used for mental conditions, Ledum Palustre can be beneficial in reducing irritability or restlessness that often accompanies physical discomfort, particularly in puncture wounds or skin irritations.

• Emotional: Emotionally, this remedy addresses the reactions to physical pain, especially pain associated with puncture wounds or insect bites. It helps in managing the emotional responses to such injuries.

• Psychological: Psychologically, Ledum Palustre aids in coping with the stress or discomfort resulting from minor injuries or skin conditions. It offers support in dealing with the psychological impact of these physical irritations.

• Physical: Known for treating puncture wounds and insect bites effectively, Ledum Palustre is also used when the affected area feels cold but is relieved by cold applications. It is particularly beneficial in managing the symptoms of these specific types of injuries.

Ledum Palustre is notable for its application in managing conditions involving puncture wounds, insect bites, and certain skin irritations, with implications for physical well-being and potential impacts on mental and emotional states.

Magnesia Phosphorica

• Mental: While Magnesia Phosphorica is not directly known for mental health applications, it can effectively reduce mental discomfort or stress that often accompanies nerve pain or muscular cramps, aiding in the alleviation of related cognitive disturbances.

• Emotional: This remedy addresses emotional responses such as distress or irritability that are common in individuals suffering from muscle cramps and nerve pain. It helps in stabilizing the emotional upheavals caused by such physical discomfort.

• Psychological: Psychologically, Magnesia Phosphorica assists in managing the stress and psychological discomfort resulting from neuromuscular issues, offering support in coping with the mental aspects of these physical conditions.

- Physical: Renowned for treating cramps, spasms, and nerve-related pains effectively, Magnesia Phosphorica is particularly beneficial in conditions like intense menstrual cramps and neuralgic pains. It plays a crucial role in alleviating the physical symptoms associated with these neuromuscular issues.

Mercurius Solubilis

• Mental: Mercurius Solubilis is extensively used for complex mental symptoms like profound restlessness and significant memory disturbances. It's particularly effective in cases related to infections or inflammatory disorders, addressing the cognitive and psychological aspects of these medical conditions.

• Emotional: This remedy plays a crucial role in managing profound emotional instability and severe mood swings, often associated with chronic infections or long-standing health issues. It aids in providing emotional balance and reducing mood variability linked to illness.

• Psychological: Psychologically, Mercurius Solubilis supports individuals dealing with the ongoing stress or anxiety of chronic health problems, offering relief from the psychological burden of enduring illness.

• Physical: Notably effective in treating a wide range of infections characterized by pronounced symptoms like excessive salivation, swollen glands, and intense night sweats, Mercurius Solubilis is also recognized for its role in addressing dental and throat infections and other related physical ailments.

This expanded insight into Mercurius Solubilis offers a detailed perspective on its application across various health conditions, focusing on its comprehensive impact on mental, emotional, psychological, and physical aspects, particularly in the context of infections and inflammatory disorders.

Natrum Muriaticum

• Mental: Natrum Muriaticum is widely used for conditions like depression, introversion, and grief, especially when these mental states are linked to past emotional trauma or heartbreak. It addresses deep-seated mental requirements like prolonged sadness and a tendency to dwell on past grievances.

• Emotional: This remedy is effective in managing emotional states characterized by reservedness and a reluctance to share feelings, often seen in individuals who have been hurt emotionally. It assists in alleviating the emotional weight of suppressed emotions and past emotional wounds.

• Psychological: Psychologically, Natrum Muriaticum aids individuals struggling with internalized grief and psychological scars from past experiences. It supports the process of emotional healing and the psychological recovery from emotional traumas.

• Physical: Known for its effectiveness in treating conditions like headaches, allergies, and skin disorders that can be exacerbated by emotional stress, Natrum Muriaticum is also used for physical symptoms related to stress and emotional upheaval.

Natrum Muriaticum is particularly notable for its application in conditions involving deep emotional issues and their physical manifestations, impacting mental, emotional, psychological, and physical health.

Nux Vomica

• Mental: Nux Vomica is significantly used for addressing mental conditions like heightened irritability, chronic impatience, and stress, particularly prevalent in highly competitive or ambitious individuals. It targets mental exhaustion and overexertion stemming from intense professional or personal demands.

• Emotional: Emotionally, this remedy is crucial in managing acute anger and frustration, commonly seen in individuals prone to perfectionism or workaholism. It aids in mitigating these strong emotional reactions and restoring dynamic equilibrium.

• Psychological: Psychologically, Nux Vomica relieves individuals overwhelmed by the stress of demanding careers or lifestyles. It supports coping with the psychological aspects of high-pressure environments and constant achievement.

• Physical: Renowned for its effectiveness in digestive ailments like indigestion, constipation, and symptoms of overindulgence, Nux Vomica is also beneficial in treating headaches and sleep disturbances related to lifestyle stress.

Nux Vomica's wide-ranging effects make it a vital remedy for conditions related to stress, lifestyle pressures, digestive issues, and associated mental, emotional, and psychological impacts.

Phosphorus

• Mental: Phosphorus is extensively used for treating mental symptoms like pervasive anxiety and pronounced fearfulness, particularly concerning the future or in social contexts. It addresses cognitive aspects of concern and helps manage the mental strain associated with social interactions or future uncertainties.

• Emotional: Emotionally, this remedy effectively balances heightened emotional sensitivity. It benefits individuals who exhibit strong empathy and compassion but may become vulnerable due to these traits. Phosphorus aids in managing emotional vulnerability and stabilizing mood swings.

• Psychological: Psychologically, Phosphorus assists in coping with the stress and emotional overwhelm that often accompany high sensitivity to others' emotions and environmental stimuli. It provides support for those who are psychologically impacted by their heightened empathic nature.

• Physical: Known for its efficacy in respiratory conditions, bleeding disorders, and nerve-related issues, Phosphorus is also used for gastrointestinal complaints and maintaining bone health. Its broad spectrum of physical applications makes it a versatile remedy for diverse medical conditions.

Pulsatilla

• Mental: Pulsatilla is widely used for mental states marked by moodiness, a tendency towards weepiness, and emotional sensitivity, especially suited for individuals with gentle, yielding personalities. It addresses the mental aspects of dynamic variability and susceptibility.

• Emotional: Emotionally, this remedy effectively manages changeable emotional states, including a pronounced need for comfort and reassurance. It's constructive for individuals who feel emotionally better with consolation and support.

• Psychological: Psychologically, Pulsatilla assists in coping with feelings of vulnerability and dependency, offering support in times of emotional overwhelm and sensitivity.

• Physical: Recognized for treating fluctuating symptoms, Pulsatilla is beneficial for menstrual disorders, digestive issues, and colds characterized by thick, changeable discharge. Its adaptability to changing physical symptoms makes it a versatile remedy.

Rhus Toxicodendron

• Mental: Rhus Toxicodendron is frequently utilized for symptoms of restlessness and anxiety, particularly when these mental states are associated with physical ailments or discomfort. It addresses the mental unease and agitation that can accompany musculoskeletal conditions.

• Emotional: This remedy effectively manages emotional agitation and irritability, often exacerbated during physical illness or pain. It aids in stabilizing emotional responses related to physical health challenges.

• Psychological: Psychologically, Rhus Toxicodendron assists in coping with the stress or frustration commonly associated with chronic pain or mobility issues, offering support for the psychological aspects of these conditions.

• Physical: Known for its effectiveness in treating musculoskeletal conditions involving joint pain, stiffness, and associated skin rashes, Rhus Toxicodendron is particularly beneficial for symptoms that improve with movement, such as those seen in rheumatic conditions.

Sepia

• Mental: Sepia is commonly used for mental states such as indifference, often towards family responsibilities or daily tasks, and is beneficial in cases of mild depression or emotional detachment. It targets the mental fatigue and lack of interest that can be prevalent in hormonal imbalances or during periods of stress.

• Emotional: This remedy addresses emotional symptoms like irritability, pronounced mood swings, and feeling overwhelmed, which are frequently related to hormonal changes. It helps in stabilizing these emotional fluctuations.

• Psychological: Psychologically, Sepia assists in managing the stress and strain of handling multiple responsibilities, particularly resonating with women who juggle personal, familial, and professional roles.

• Physical: Known for treating hormonal imbalances, menstrual disorders, and menopausal symptoms, Sepia is also effective for chronic fatigue and reproductive system-related conditions. Its application extends to a range of gynecological and hormonal health issues.

Silicea

• Mental: Silicea is widely used for treating conditions like lack of self-confidence, indecision, and nervousness, especially when facing challenges. It addresses the mental aspects of insecurity and hesitation, which are often beneficial for individuals who struggle with assertiveness and decision-making.

• Emotional: This remedy effectively manages emotional fragility and sensitivity, which are common in individuals easily overwhelmed by stress or conflict. It assists in balancing emotional responses and enhancing emotional resilience.

• Psychological: Psychologically, Silicea supports individuals dealing with feelings of vulnerability and the psychological impacts of stress, providing relief in managing these mental burdens.

• Physical: Recognized for its effectiveness in improving the health of skin, hair, and nails, Silicea is also beneficial in conditions involving connective tissues and bones. It aids in the body's natural process of expelling foreign bodies from the skin.

Silicea's comprehensive application extends to improving connective tissue strength, enhancing skin, hair, and nail health, and offering benefits for mental and emotional well-being.

Staphysagria

• Mental: Staphysagria is extensively utilized for conditions linked to suppressed emotions or unresolved anger. It is particularly effective in cases where such feelings are internalized, leading to mental and emotional strain. It addresses the mental repercussions of harboring unresolved emotional issues.

• Emotional: This remedy is adept at managing emotional sensitivity, deep-seated resentment, and frustration, commonly stemming from feelings of being wronged or insulted. It assists individuals in processing and releasing these emotional burdens.

• Psychological: Psychologically, Staphysagria supports individuals in coping with suppressed anger and addressing emotional wounds. It aids in the psychological healing process, particularly for those who have internalized their emotional pain.

• Physical: Known for treating conditions that arise from suppressed emotions, like skin eruptions or urinary tract issues, Staphysagria is also beneficial in post-surgical recovery or after experiencing physical trauma.

Staphysagria's role extends to managing the physical manifestations of suppressed emotions and aiding in the recovery of both mental and emotional health, making it a significant remedy in holistic care.

Sulfur

• Mental: Sulphur enhances intellectual curiosity while addressing mental restlessness and deep philosophical contemplation. It benefits individuals with a tendency toward constant mental activity, often leading to mental overstimulation and fatigue.

• Emotional: On an emotional level, Sulphur assists in moderating irritability and a predisposition to be overly critical or opinionated. It helps in balancing these emotional tendencies, reducing judgmental attitudes, and fostering a more tolerant emotional outlook.

• Psychological: Psychologically, Sulphur is vital in managing the stress and anxiety associated with continuous mental activity and the inclination to overanalyze. It supports individuals in dealing with the psychological consequences of an overactive mental process.

- Physical: Renowned for its effectiveness in various physical conditions, Sulphur is especially beneficial in treating skin conditions, chronic inflammations, and circulatory issues. It is also known for its detoxifying effects on the body, promoting overall physical health and aiding in systemic purification.

Sulfur's extensive application in homeopathy makes it a fundamental remedy, impacting a wide range of mental, emotional, psychological, and physical health aspects. Its versatility and broad-spectrum efficacy underscore its quintessential role in homeopathic treatment.

Veratrum Album

- Mental: Veratrum Album is profoundly effective in treating acute mental conditions such as intense fear, delusions, and severe despair. It's particularly beneficial when these symptoms are acute, marked by extreme intensity and sudden onset.

- Emotional: This remedy is critical in managing deep emotional turmoil. It addresses severe mood swings, hysteria, and tendencies towards deep melancholy or despair, making it essential in acute emotional crises.

- Psychological: Psychologically, the Veratrum Album assists in coping with extreme psychological states, including severe anxiety, panic attacks, and acute stress reactions. It offers significant support in managing these intense psychological symptoms.

- Physical: Known for its efficacy in treating severe acute conditions like profuse vomiting, diarrhea, and states of collapse, Veratrum Album is also used in cases characterized by profound weakness and dehydration.

Antimonium Tartaricum

• Mental: Antimonium Tartaricum is widely utilized for treating mental symptoms such as irritability and a sense of discontent, particularly in individuals feeling physically weak or debilitated. It's effective in cases where physical ailment leads to mental irritability and dissatisfaction.

• Emotional: Emotionally, this remedy is beneficial in addressing states of restlessness or frustration, especially in those prone to agitation. It helps manage emotional responses in individuals who are easily disturbed or upset.

• Psychological: Psychologically, Antimonium Tartaricum assists individuals who struggle with the mental effects of physical weakness or illness. It supports the coping mechanisms for dealing with the psychological impact of health-related issues.

• Physical: Known for its efficacy in respiratory conditions like coughs with significant mucus congestion, Antimonium Tartaricum is also used for various digestive disturbances. It is particularly beneficial for respiratory and digestive symptoms where there is a need to expel mucus or other congestive substances.

Aurum Metallicum

• Mental: Aurum Metallicum is extensively used for severe depression and profound feelings of despair, particularly related to a deep sense of personal failure or guilt. It addresses the psychological depths of pain when an individual feels they have not met their or others' expectations.

• Emotional: This remedy is crucial in managing intense emotional states like deep sadness and self-reproach. It is often chosen in cases where there are severe feelings of worthlessness and, in extreme cases, suicidal thoughts, usually stemming from perceived personal failures or acute disappointments.

• Psychological: Psychologically, Aurum Metallicum is instrumental in coping with the mental anguish associated with high personal standards and self-criticism. It supports individuals who place immense pressure on themselves and struggle with the psychological fallout of failing to meet these standards.

• Physical: Known for its effectiveness in heart-related issues, including high blood pressure and night-time palpitations, Aurum Metallicum is also used in bone health, particularly for deep-seated, bony pains. Its application extends to both cardiovascular and structural physical ailments.

Berberis Vulgaris

• Mental: While Berberis Vulgaris is not primarily used for direct mental effects, it can be beneficial in alleviating mental discomfort or irritability often associated with physical ailments, particularly urinary and renal conditions. It helps to reduce the mental frustration that can accompany chronic physical disorders.

• Emotional: This remedy addresses emotional reactions like frustration or impatience, especially related to enduring physical health issues. It aids in managing emotional responses to persistent discomfort and pain.

• Psychological: Psychologically, Berberis Vulgaris is effective for those experiencing the stress or psychological strain of ongoing health concerns, particularly those related to the urinary and renal systems.

• Physical: Renowned for its efficacy in treating kidney and urinary tract conditions, including kidney stones and urinary discomfort, Berberis Vulgaris is also beneficial for addressing joint and back pain, often related to its primary action on the renal system.

Calcarea Phosphorica

- Mental: Calcarea Phosphorica is widely used for mental symptoms like difficulty concentrating, fatigue, and confusion. It's particularly beneficial for individuals, including adolescents, who experience cognitive fatigue or lack of focus, often related to growth or developmental stages.

- Emotional: This remedy addresses emotional states such as discontent and a strong desire for change, frequently seen in adolescents or during periods of significant growth and development. It helps in managing the emotional upheavals associated with these transitional phases.

- Psychological: Psychologically, Calcarea Phosphorica aids individuals feeling overwhelmed by life transitions, growth challenges, or developmental changes, providing support in coping with these psychological aspects.

- Physical: Known for its efficacy in treating issues related to bones and teeth, primarily during growth periods in children, Calcarea Phosphorica is also used for joint pains and digestive-specific problems. It plays a crucial role in supporting physical development and addressing growth-related ailments.

Calcarea Sulphurica

- Mental: While not directly impacting mental health, Calcarea Sulphurica can alleviate irritability or restlessness that often accompanies chronic physical conditions, particularly skin ailments. It helps in reducing the mental discomfort associated with ongoing physical issues.

- Emotional: This remedy addresses emotional responses, such as frustration or discomfort, that arise from skin conditions or persistent infections. It assists in managing the emotional distress related to these physical ailments.

- Psychological: Psychologically, Calcarea Sulphurica benefits those dealing with the stress and psychological impact of continuous physical conditions, especially those involving skin health.
- Physical: Calcarea Sulphurica is known for effectively treating various skin conditions, including abscesses, pimples, and wounds that are slow to heal. It is beneficial in cases where purulent discharges, aiding in the healing process and recovery of skin health.

Carcinosin

- Mental: Carcinosin is often used for deep-seated anxiety, particularly when it relates to personal or family health history. It addresses mental stress and worry that can arise in individuals with a significant history of familial diseases.
- Emotional: This remedy is effective in managing emotional depth and sensitivity, commonly found in individuals who have a strong family history of chronic illnesses, including cancer. It helps in balancing emotional responses linked to genetic predispositions.
- Psychological: Psychologically, Carcinosin aids in coping with the stress and concern associated with genetic predispositions or a family history of severe health conditions. It supports individuals dealing with the psychological aspects of such health concerns.
- Physical: Known for its application in cases with a strong familial history of cancer, Carcinosin is also used for various conditions based on individual symptomatology and constitutional factors. It is considered particularly when there is a significant medical history of cancer in the family.

Carcinosin's comprehensive application highlights its role in treating individuals with significant family health histories, affecting mental, emotional, psychological, and physical health, particularly in the context of familial disease predispositions.

Caulophyllum

• Mental: While Caulophyllum is not primarily focused on mental symptoms, it can be supportive in alleviating mental stress, particularly when related to menstrual issues or the process of childbirth. It helps manage the mental aspects of gynecological health, such as stress or worry.

• Emotional: Emotionally, this remedy helps address the fluctuations often associated with menstrual cycles or childbirth. It assists in stabilizing emotional responses and helps manage mood swings related to hormonal changes.

• Psychological: Psychologically, Caulophyllum aids in coping with stress and anxiety, especially those linked to gynecological health or childbirth. It offers support to women dealing with the psychological impact of menstrual disorders or labor difficulties.

• Physical: Known for treating menstrual disorders, difficulties during labor, and joint pains, particularly in the small joints. It's effective in easing menstrual cramps irregular cycles, and assisting with childbirth-related issues.

Chelidonium Majus

• Mental: While Chelidonium Majus is not primarily used for mental health, it can be effective in alleviating irritability or mood changes often associated with liver-related issues. It addresses the mental and emotional disturbances that can arise from liver dysfunction.

• Emotional: Emotionally, this remedy is beneficial in managing disturbances that may stem from liver or digestive system problems. It helps in stabilizing emotional responses related to physical health issues.

• Psychological: Psychologically, Chelidonium Majus aids individuals coping with the stress or discomfort caused by chronic conditions of the liver or gallbladder, offering support in dealing with the psychological aspects of these health issues.

• Physical: Known for treating liver and gallbladder disorders, Chelidonium Majus is also used for various digestive issues and conditions that specifically affect the right side of the body. Its role in enhancing liver function and addressing related health concerns is significant.

Cinchona Officinalis (China)

• Mental: Cinchona Officinalis is highly effective for mental fatigue and cognitive weakness, especially following the significant loss of bodily fluids or enduring chronic illness. It's particularly beneficial in improving mental clarity and reducing fatigue associated with physical debilitation.

• Emotional: This remedy is crucial in addressing emotional sensitivity and irritability that may be heightened during physical weakness or recovery from illness. It assists in stabilizing emotional fluctuations during convalescence.

• Psychological: Psychologically, Cinchona Officinalis supports individuals feeling psychologically drained or overwhelmed due to physical weakness, aiding in the recovery of psychological resilience post-illness.

• Physical: Known for its efficacy in treating conditions caused by loss of bodily fluids, such as bleeding, severe diarrhea, or profuse sweating, China is also recognized for its therapeutic properties in combating weakness and fatigue. It is a crucial remedy in rejuvenating the body post-fluid loss or in cases of chronic debilitation.

Crotalus Horridus

• Mental: Crotalus Horridus is notably used for treating mental confusion and disorientation, especially in severe illness or toxic states. It addresses cognitive impairments that arise in the context of significant health challenges, including encephalopathy and severe systemic infections.

• Emotional: This remedy aids in managing emotional instability and pronounced mood swings, which are often observed in individuals dealing with severe or life-threatening health conditions. It helps to stabilize emotional fluctuations under these stressful circumstances.

• Psychological: Psychologically, Crotalus Horridus is beneficial in coping with the stress, anxiety, and fear associated with severe health conditions, including septic states and life-threatening infections.

• Physical: Recognized for its effectiveness in treating hemorrhagic conditions, blood disorders, and severe infections, Crotalus Horridus is used in cases involving septicemia and other painful health crises. It is vital in managing physical symptoms associated with blood toxicity and systemic conditions.

Cuprum Metallicum

• Mental: Cuprum Metallicum is used extensively for treating mental rigidity and symptoms associated with neurological disorders, including spasmodic conditions. It addresses the mental strain and cognitive issues that can arise from neuromuscular diseases.

• Emotional: This remedy is effective in managing intense emotional reactions like fear or anxiety, often triggered by physical symptoms such as cramps or spasms. It helps in stabilizing emotional responses to such physical conditions.

- Psychological: Psychologically, Cuprum Metallicum aids individuals in coping with the stress or trauma associated with convulsive disorders or muscular spasms. It offers support in dealing with the psychological impact of these conditions.

- Physical: Recognized for its effectiveness in treating muscle spasms, cramps, and various convulsive disorders, Cuprum Metallicum is also used in respiratory conditions like asthma and bronchitis, with prominent spasmodic symptoms.

Digitalis Purpurea

- Mental: While Digitalis Purpurea is not primarily known for mental effects, it can be effective in reducing anxiety specifically related to heart conditions. This remedy can aid in alleviating the mental worry and apprehension that often accompany cardiac issues.

- Emotional: This remedy addresses emotional responses linked to the fear of heart disease, palpitations, or other heart-related anxieties. It helps in stabilizing emotional reactions associated with concerns over cardiac health.

- Psychological: Psychologically, Digitalis Purpurea is beneficial in managing the stress or anxiety that may arise from concerns about cardiac health, including conditions like arrhythmias or heart failure.

- Physical: Recognized for its effectiveness in treating various heart conditions, Digitalis Purpurea is mainly used in cases with specific symptoms such as arrhythmias, heart failure, and palpitations. It plays a crucial role in managing the physical symptoms of these cardiac conditions.

Echinacea Angustifolia

- Mental: While not directly targeting mental health, Echinacea Angustifolia can indirectly support mental well-being by improving overall physical health. This support can lead to better mental clarity and reduced stress related to health concerns.

• Emotional: This remedy enhances emotional resilience, which is especially beneficial for individuals with weakened immune systems or those prone to frequent infections. It assists in fostering a sense of emotional strength and stability.

• Psychological: Psychologically, Echinacea Angustifolia effectively manages stress associated with ongoing health issues or illness susceptibility. It helps individuals cope with the psychological aspects of maintaining health.

• Physical: Known for its effectiveness in boosting immune function, Echinacea Angustifolia is widely used in treating recurrent infections, aiding wound healing, and promoting general health. It's an essential remedy for enhancing the body's natural defense mechanisms.

The following remedy for detailed analysis is Graphites. Here's an extensive overview:

Graphites

• Mental: Graphites are often used for individuals experiencing mild depression or indecision, particularly when these mental states are associated with skin conditions or metabolic imbalances.

• Emotional: This remedy addresses emotional sensitivity and a propensity towards melancholy, especially in those who struggle with chronic skin issues or weight problems.

• Psychological: Psychologically, Graphites can aid in managing the stress or anxiety related to persistent health concerns, such as skin disorders or metabolic disturbances.

• Physical: Known for its effectiveness in treating skin conditions like eczema, psoriasis, and dry skin, Graphites is also used for metabolic issues like obesity and constipation.

Graphites are particularly noted for their application in conditions involving skin and metabolic issues, impacting mental, emotional, psychological, and physical health.

Hamamelis Virginiana
• Mental: While Hamamelis Virginiana is not primarily focused on mental health, it can be supportive in reducing irritability or discomfort associated with circulatory issues. This can indirectly alleviate mental stress linked to physical conditions involving the veins.

• Emotional: This remedy aids in managing emotional distress related to venous conditions. It benefits individuals experiencing emotional responses due to physical discomfort from conditions like varicose veins or hemorrhoids.

• Psychological: Psychologically, Hamamelis Virginiana assists those dealing with the stress or psychological strain of venous disorders, offering support in managing the psychological impact of these conditions.

• Physical: Recognized for its effectiveness in treating venous system disorders, Hamamelis Virginiana is extensively used for conditions like varicose veins, hemorrhoids, and bruising. It addresses symptoms of venous congestion and bleeding, making it an essential remedy in treating venous health issues.

You might also be interested in the following Materia Medica's

"Kent's New Repertory" by James Tyler Kent is a cornerstone of homeopathic literature. Kent's meticulous work offers a comprehensive repertory, serving as a guide to symptomatology and remedy selection. With its systematic approach and cross-referencing, this repertory aids practitioners in finding the most fitting remedies for various conditions.

Boericke's Materia Medica by William Boericke

"Boericke's Materia Medica" by William Boericke is a classic work that presents remedies in a concise and accessible format. Boericke's insights provide characteristic symptoms and keynotes for each remedy, allowing for quick reference and understanding. This materia medica is a valuable tool for both beginners and experienced practitioners.

Hering's Guiding Symptoms of Our Materia Medica by Constantine Hering

"Hering's Guiding Symptoms of Our Materia Medica" by Constantine Hering is a seminal contribution to homeopathic literature. Hering's emphasis on the direction of cure and symptom progression guides practitioners in understanding the dynamic nature of healing. This work provides a deep exploration of remedies and their effects over time.

Synoptic Key to Materia Medica by Cyrus Maxwell Boger

"Synoptic Key to Materia Medica" by Cyrus Maxwell Boger is revered for synthesizing keynotes and characteristics. Boger's unique approach aids in distinguishing between closely related remedies. This work simplifies remedy differentiation, making it an invaluable support in accurate prescribing.

"Leaders in Homeopathic Therapeutics" by E.B. Nash is a practical guide to therapeutics, offering insights into remedy selection for specific conditions. Nash's clinical experience shines as he discusses indications, modalities, and case examples. This work empowers practitioners with actionable information for effective treatment.

Allen's Keynotes and Characteristics by Henry Clay Allen

"Allen's Keynotes and Characteristics" by Henry Clay Allen presents characteristic symptoms and keynotes of remedies. Allen's concise and insightful descriptions aid practitioners in quickly recognizing the essence of each treatment. This work is a valuable reference for understanding remedy profiles.

Vermeulen's Concordant Materia Medica by Frans Vermeulen

"Vermeulen's Concordant Materia Medica" by Frans Vermeulen offers a fresh perspective on remedies, drawing connections between materia medica sources. Vermeulen's meticulous research highlights remedy relationships, expanding our understanding of their interconnectedness.

Murphy's Clinical Materia Medica by Robin Murphy

"Murphy's Clinical Materia Medica" by Robin Murphy is a modern compendium that integrates traditional symptomatology with contemporary insights. Murphy's work bridges the gap between classical and modern approaches, providing a comprehensive view of remedy indications.

Phatak's Materia Medica by S.R. Phatak

"Phatak's Materia Medica" by S.R. Phatak is known for its practical approach, offering insights into common and rare remedies. Phatak's work includes clinical experiences and case examples, making it a valuable guide for day-to-day practice.

The Twelve Tissue Remedies of Schüssler by Boericke and Dewey

"The Twelve Tissue Remedies of Schüssler" by Boericke and Dewey delves into tissue salts, providing insights into their therapeutic applications. This work offers a unique perspective on remedies that address cellular imbalances.

A Study on Materia Medica by N. M. Choudhuri

"A Study on Materia Medica" by N. M. Choudhuri is a comprehensive exploration of remedies, emphasizing their psychological and emotional aspects. Choudhuri's work enriches our understanding of remedies beyond the physical realm.

Encyclopedia of Pure Materia Medica by Timothy Field Allen

"Encyclopedia of Pure Materia Medica" by Timothy Field Allen is a monumental work that presents exhaustive details of remedies. Allen's meticulous approach provides a deep dive into remedy sources and their effects on various dimensions of health.

These presentations provide a glimpse into the contributions and unique perspectives offered by each of these materia medica books, empowering practitioners with a wealth of knowledge for effective homeopathic practice

In conclusion:

Concluding the chapter on Materia Medica allows us to consolidate the extensive insights we have garnered regarding medicinal substances and their therapeutic applications. This chapter is a pivotal foundation for understanding the pharmacological attributes and historical context of various agents derived from botanical, mineral, and animal sources.

Throughout our exploration of Materia Medica, we have delved into the fundamental principles that underpin the selection and utilization of various remedies. The significance of provings, experiments, and systematic observations has underscored the empirical nature of this study. These practices are essential not only for substantiating the effects of substances but also for refining our understanding of their nuances in different clinical scenarios.

Historical dimensions have lent depth to our comprehension of Materia Medica. The journey has revealed the enduring influence of traditional remedies on modern medical practices. By tracing the evolution of materia medica across cultures and eras, we have recognized the adaptability of these remedies, as well as their incorporation into contemporary healthcare frameworks. This historical contextualization aids us in appreciating the dynamic nature of medicinal substances.

A cornerstone of Materia Medica is meticulous observation and documentation. Practitioners and researchers have meticulously recorded the symptoms, reactions, and outcomes associated with various substances. This empirical evidence is pivotal in unraveling the intricacies of each remedy's therapeutic potential. These documented experiences constitute a valuable repository of knowledge that informs clinical decision-making.

As we transition from this chapter, we must acknowledge the symbiotic relationship between tradition and progress. While rooted in historical wisdom, Materia Medica is not static. The intersection of traditional understanding with modern scientific inquiry has shed light on the molecular mechanisms that govern the interactions between medicinal agents and the human body. This integration enriches our experience and paves the way for evidence-based integration into contemporary medical paradigms.

In conclusion, the chapter on Materia Medica extends an invitation to a lifelong journey of exploration. The foundation laid here equips us with the tools to select remedies judiciously, considering their historical significance, empirical evidence, and emerging scientific insights. The chapter encapsulates the essence of the healing arts—a harmonious amalgamation of ancient wisdom, rigorous observation, and scientific inquiry. As we advance, these insights accompany us, enriching our practice and fostering our commitment to the well-being of those under our care.

Chapter 3: An inquiry into men's and women's health issues

In this groundbreaking chapter, we embark on a comprehensive journey of exploration, shedding light on the often overlooked and crucial domain of women's and men's health issues. As we delve deep into the intricate web of medical complexities faced by individuals of all genders, we aim to provide an even more in-depth and exhaustive understanding of the diverse health challenges that impact women and men equally.

The significance of gender-specific healthcare cannot be overstated, as women and men experience distinct physiological, hormonal, and genetic differences throughout their lives. Women's health issues encompass a vast array of conditions, ranging from reproductive health concerns, such as menstrual irregularities, polycystic ovarian syndrome (PCOS), and endometriosis, to pregnancy-related complications and menopausal symptoms. Additionally, we delve into the intricacies of breast health, gynecological cancers, and autoimmune diseases that disproportionately affect women.

Similarly, men's health issues merit equal attention, exploring topics such as prostate health, male infertility, and testicular conditions. We also address cardiovascular health, mental health, and the impact of hormonal changes, providing comprehensive insights into the unique challenges men encounter in different stages of life.

Within the pages of this chapter, you will find a diverse array of health conditions affecting individuals of all sexes, all meticulously researched and presented. We aim to empower readers to make informed decisions about their health by equipping them with an even more comprehensive range of treatment options. While conventional medicine plays a critical role in healthcare, we also recognize the value of exploring homeopathic and alternative remedies, as they can provide viable and complementary approaches to managing various conditions for both women and men.

Through an evidence-based approach, we endeavor to dispel myths, debunk misconceptions, and present an unbiased view of the efficacy of different treatments for everyone. Our commitment to accuracy and thoroughness ensures that readers find a wealth of knowledge, fostering an environment where individuals of all genders can actively participate in their healthcare decisions.

Moreover, as we traverse through this chapter, we must not lose sight of the societal and cultural factors that influence health outcomes. Addressing disparities, access to healthcare, and understanding the impact of gender norms on health-seeking behaviors are all critical aspects of our exploration of everyone's health and well-being.

In conclusion, this extensive and informative chapter aims to be a guiding light, illuminating the path toward better health and well-being for all, regardless of gender. By embracing a holistic and inclusive perspective, we envision a future where individuals of all sexes can navigate their health journeys with empowerment, knowledge, and compassion.

The best aspects of a woman. In celebration of womanhood.

Empathy: One of the most admirable traits in a woman is her profound empathy. She has the innate ability to understand and share the feelings of others, making her a compassionate and caring presence in people's lives. Her capacity for empathy allows her to connect with others on a deep emotional level, offering comfort and support in times of need.

Resilience: A remarkable attribute of a woman is her resilience. She faces life's challenges with unwavering strength and determination. No matter the obstacles that come her way, she bounces back with courage, learning from experiences and using them to grow stronger and more confident.

Nurturing: The nurturing nature of a woman is a beautiful aspect of her character. Whether as a mother, caregiver, or friend, she provides unwavering care and support to those around her. Her nurturing instincts create a safe and loving environment where people feel valued and cherished.

Intelligence: A woman's intelligence is a powerful asset. She possesses a diverse range of intellectual abilities and excels in various fields of knowledge. Her thirst for learning drives her to explore new ideas, contributing to advancements in science, arts, technology, and more.

Emotional Intelligence: The emotional intelligence of a woman is genuinely commendable. She possesses an acute understanding of emotions, both in herself and others. This enables her to communicate effectively, navigate complex social situations with finesse, and build solid and meaningful relationships.

Creativity: A woman's imagination knows no bounds. She brings unique perspectives and innovative ideas to the forefront. Whether it's through art, problem-solving, or imaginative thinking, her creativity enriches the world and inspires those around her.

Empowerment: Empowering herself and others is a fundamental aspect of a woman's character. She is a source of inspiration, advocating for equality and justice and uplifting those who need support. Her drive for positive change leaves a lasting impact on her community and beyond.

Adaptability: A woman's adaptability is commendable. She thrives in diverse environments and embraces change with grace. Her ability to adjust to new circumstances and remain open to different perspectives allows her to grow and evolve continually.

Intuition: A woman's intuition is a valuable asset in decision-making and navigating life's complexities. She possesses a keen sense of insight, guiding her towards making thoughtful and insightful choices.

Leadership: Many women are natural leaders. Their strong organizational skills and ability to motivate and inspire others make them influential leaders. They prioritize teamwork and collaboration, fostering an inclusive and supportive environment.

Patience: A woman's patience and understanding create a harmonious interaction atmosphere. She approaches challenges and conflicts calmly, seeking wisdom and resolution rather than haste.

Diplomacy: Women often excel in diplomacy, skillfully navigating conflicts and negotiations with empathy and tact. They prioritize open communication and strive for win-win solutions in any situation.

Respecting Diversity: Embracing diversity is a core value for women. They celebrate different cultures, backgrounds, and perspectives, fostering an inclusive environment where everyone feels valued and respected.

Humility: Despite their achievements, many women remain humble and down-to-earth. They value collective efforts and teamwork, recognizing that individual successes are often a result of the support of others.

Courage: A woman's courage and fearlessness are commendable. She stands up for her beliefs and principles, even when faced with challenges or opposition. Her determination to bring about positive change is truly inspiring.

Ambition: Driven by ambition, women pursue their goals passionately and passionately. They continuously strive for personal growth and excellence in their lives.

Social Awareness: Women possess a keen sense of social issues and actively engage in community initiatives. They use their voice to advocate for causes close to their hearts, working towards positively impacting society.

Generosity: The generosity of women knows no bounds. They are selfless in offering their time, resources, and compassion to help others in need, making a significant difference in the lives of those they touch.

Sense of Community: Women foster a strong sense of community and support wherever they go. They build meaningful relationships and create networks of mutual support and encouragement.

Sense of Humor: Women's sense of humor brings joy and laughter to those around them. Their ability to find humor in various situations creates a positive and enjoyable atmosphere in their interactions.

Curiosity: Women's insatiable curiosity drives them to explore and seek knowledge about the world around them. They approach learning with enthusiasm, continually expanding their horizons.

Open-Mindedness: Women are open to new ideas and perspectives, embracing diversity and valuing the insights of others. Their open-mindedness fosters a spirit of collaboration and mutual understanding.

Gratitude: Women express gratitude and appreciation for the positive aspects of life. They recognize and cherish the blessings they receive, fostering a sense of contentment and mindfulness.

Integrity: Guided by strong moral principles and ethics, women uphold integrity in all aspects of their lives. Their honesty and authenticity earn them the trust and respect of those around them.

Spirituality: Women explore and find solace in their spiritual beliefs, enriching their lives with a sense of purpose and inner peace.

These attributes showcase the diverse and admirable qualities that women possess, making them truly remarkable and inspiring individuals.

Here are some considerations that deal specifically with women's health issues

Disclaimer: The information provided is for entertainment purposes only. This is not to be considered medical advice in any way.

If you are experiencing any of these symptoms, please see a licensed, qualified healthcare practitioner.

Some frequent health issues address women's concerns.

Menstrual disorders:

Menstrual disorders refer to a range of conditions that affect a woman's menstrual cycle. This can include irregular periods, heavy bleeding (menorrhagia), prolonged periods (menometrorrhagia), or the absence of menstruation (amenorrhea). These disorders can be caused by various factors, such as hormonal imbalances, thyroid issues, polycystic ovary syndrome (PCOS), or uterine abnormalities. They can impact a woman's physical and emotional well-being, and treatment options may include hormonal medications, lifestyle changes, or surgical interventions.

Polycystic Ovary Syndrome (PCOS):

PCOS is a hormonal disorder that affects the ovaries. It is characterized by enlarged ovaries containing small cysts. Women with PCOS may experience irregular or absent periods, excess hair growth (hirsutism), acne, weight gain, and fertility issues. PCOS is caused by hormonal imbalances, specifically elevated levels of androgens (male hormones) and insulin resistance. Treatment focuses on managing symptoms and may involve lifestyle modifications, hormonal contraceptives, and medications to regulate menstrual cycles and control other symptoms.

Endometriosis:

Endometriosis is a condition where tissue similar to the lining of the uterus grows outside the uterus. This can cause pain, particularly during menstruation, pelvic discomfort, heavy or irregular periods, and fertility problems. The displaced tissue can adhere to other organs in the pelvic area, forming adhesions and causing inflammation. The exact cause of endometriosis is unknown, but it is thought to involve hormonal, genetic, and immune system factors. Treatment options range from pain management medications to hormone therapies and, in severe cases, surgical removal of endometrial tissue.

Fibroids:

Uterine fibroids are non-cancerous growths that develop in or around the uterus. They are composed of muscle and connective tissue. Fibroids can vary in size and number and may cause symptoms such as heavy or prolonged menstrual bleeding, pelvic pressure, frequent urination, and pain during intercourse. The exact cause of fibroids is unclear, but hormonal factors influence them. Treatment options include medication to manage symptoms, hormonal therapies to shrink the fibroids, or surgery to remove them.

Vaginal infections:

Vaginal infections are caused by an overgrowth of bacteria, fungi, or viruses in the vaginal area. Common types of vaginal infections include yeast infections (caused by Candida overgrowth), bacterial vaginosis (resulting from an imbalance of vaginal bacteria), and sexually transmitted infections (STIs) such as chlamydia, gonorrhea, or trichomoniasis. Symptoms can include abnormal vaginal discharge, itching, burning, and discomfort during urination or intercourse. Treatment varies depending on the specific infection and may involve antifungal or antibiotic medications.

Pelvic Inflammatory Disease (PID):

PID is an infection of the female reproductive organs, typically caused by sexually transmitted bacteria such as chlamydia or gonorrhea. It can also occur due to other sources of bacterial infection. PID can lead to inflammation, scarring, and damage to the fallopian tubes, uterus, and ovaries. Symptoms may include pelvic pain, abnormal vaginal discharge, painful urination, and fever. Prompt treatment with antibiotics is essential to prevent complications and preserve fertility.

Pelvic organs prolapse:

Pelvic organ prolapse occurs when the pelvic organs, such as the uterus, bladder, or rectum, descend from their regular positions and bulge into the vaginal canal. This can be caused by weakened pelvic floor muscles and ligaments due to factors like childbirth, aging, obesity, or chronic coughing. Symptoms can range from a feeling of pelvic pressure and discomfort to urinary incontinence and difficulty emptying the bladder or bowels. Treatment options include pelvic floor exercises, pessaries (supportive devices), or surgical interventions.

Urinary incontinence:

Urinary incontinence is the involuntary loss of bladder control, resulting in urine leakage. Weakened pelvic floor muscles, nerve damage, hormonal changes, or certain medical conditions can cause it. Types of urinary incontinence include stress incontinence (leakage with physical exertion or coughing), urge incontinence (sudden strong urge to urinate), and overflow incontinence (inability to empty the bladder). Treatment options include lifestyle changes, pelvic floor exercises, medication, or surgical procedures, depending on the underlying cause.

Morning sickness:

Morning sickness refers to nausea and vomiting commonly occurring during early pregnancy, although it can affect some women throughout their pregnancy. The exact cause is unknown, but hormonal changes and increased sensitivity to certain smells and tastes are believed to contribute to its development. Symptoms typically improve as pregnancy progresses, but in severe cases, medication and lifestyle changes can help manage the symptoms.

Breast health:

Breast health encompasses various conditions related to the breast tissue, including breast pain (mastalgia), breast lumps or masses, nipple discharge, or breast abnormalities. While breast changes can be a regular part of hormonal fluctuations, specific symptoms may warrant medical attention to rule out breast cancer or other conditions. Regular breast self-exams, clinical breast exams, and mammograms are essential for monitoring breast health and detecting any abnormalities.

Postpartum depression:

Postpartum depression is a mood disorder that affects some women after giving birth. It is characterized by feelings of sadness, anxiety, exhaustion, and irritability that can interfere with daily functioning and bonding with the newborn. Postpartum depression is believed to be caused by hormonal changes, emotional stress, and other factors. Treatment may involve therapy, support groups, medication, and a robust support system to help the new mother navigate through this challenging time.

Hormonal imbalances: Hormonal imbalances can occur due to various factors, such as stress, certain medical conditions, medications, or lifestyle factors. These imbalances can manifest in a wide range of symptoms, including irregular periods, mood swings, fatigue, weight changes, acne, and changes in libido. Treatment depends on the specific hormonal imbalance and may involve lifestyle modifications, hormonal therapy, or addressing the underlying cause.

Ovarian cysts:

Ovarian cysts are fluid-filled sacs that can form on or within the ovaries. They are usually benign and often resolve on their own without causing symptoms. However, larger cysts or those that persist can lead to pelvic pain or discomfort, bloating, and changes in menstrual patterns. Treatment options range from watchful waiting to medication or surgery, depending on the size, type, and symptoms associated with the cyst.

Vulvodynia:

Vulvodynia is a chronic condition characterized by persistent pain or discomfort in the vulvar area. The exact cause is unknown, but factors such as nerve irritation, muscle spasms, hormonal changes, and previous vaginal infections or trauma may contribute to its development. Symptoms can include burning, stinging, or rawness in the vulvar region. Treatment often involves a multidisciplinary approach, including topical medications, physical therapy, counseling, and lifestyle changes to manage symptoms and improve quality of life.

Pelvic discomfort:

Pelvic discomfort refers to a range of symptoms such as pain, pressure, or discomfort in the pelvic region. It can have various causes, including menstrual disorders, pelvic inflammatory disease, endometriosis, fibroids, urinary tract infections, or musculoskeletal issues. Treatment depends on the underlying cause and may involve medications, lifestyle changes, physical therapy, or surgical interventions.

Uterine fibroids:

Uterine fibroids are non-cancerous growths that develop in the uterus. They can vary in size and location within the uterus and may cause symptoms such as heavy or prolonged menstrual bleeding, pelvic pressure, frequent urination, and pain during intercourse. The exact cause of fibroids is unknown, but hormonal factors, genetics, and family history are believed to play a role. Treatment options range from watchful waiting to medication or surgical procedures depending on the severity of symptoms and desire for fertility preservation.

Hormonal acne:

Hormonal acne refers to breakouts influenced by hormonal fluctuations, typically during puberty, the menstrual cycle, or hormonal disorders. Increased androgens (male hormones) can stimulate excess oil production in the skin, leading to clogged pores and acne. Treatment options for hormonal acne may include topical medications, oral contraceptives, anti-androgen medications, or prescription acne treatments.

Premenstrual Syndrome (PMS):

PMS refers to physical and emotional symptoms that occur in the days or weeks leading to menstruation. Common symptoms include mood swings, irritability, bloating, breast tenderness, fatigue, and food cravings. While the exact cause is unclear, hormonal changes, serotonin fluctuations, and sensitivity to progesterone and estrogen are thought to contribute. Lifestyle changes, dietary modifications, exercise, and medication can help manage PMS symptoms.

Premenstrual Dysphoric Disorder (PMDD):

PMDD is a severe form of premenstrual syndrome characterized by intense mood swings, irritability, depression, anxiety, and other emotional symptoms. These symptoms significantly impact daily functioning and relationships. The exact cause of PMDD is unknown but is believed to involve hormonal changes and neurotransmitter imbalances. Treatment options may include lifestyle changes, counseling, medications, or hormonal therapies.

Cervicitis:

Cervicitis refers to inflammation of the cervix, typically caused by an infection, such as a sexually transmitted infection (STI) or other bacterial or viral infections. Symptoms may include vaginal discharge, pain during intercourse, pelvic discomfort, and abnormal bleeding. Treatment involves identifying and treating the underlying condition with antibiotics, antiviral medications, or other appropriate therapies.

Absent menstruation (amenorrhea):

Amenorrhea is the absence of menstrual periods. Various factors, including hormonal imbalances, pregnancy, breastfeeding, extreme weight loss or gain, excessive exercise, certain medical conditions, or medications, can cause it. Treatment depends on the underlying cause and may involve lifestyle modifications, hormonal therapies, or addressing the specific situation causing amenorrhea.

Vaginismus:

Vaginismus is a condition characterized by involuntary muscle spasms in the pelvic floor muscles, making it difficult or impossible to engage in vaginal penetration. Physical or emotional factors, such as fear, anxiety, trauma, or certain medical conditions, can cause it. Treatment may involve physical therapy, counseling, gradual desensitization, or dilators to help relax the pelvic muscles and overcome the disease.

Vaginal dryness:

Vaginal dryness refers to a lack of moisture and lubrication in the vaginal area, often caused by hormonal changes, menopause, certain medications, or medical conditions. It can lead to discomfort, itching, pain during intercourse, and an increased risk of vaginal infections. Treatment options may include over-the-counter or prescription lubricants, hormone therapy, or addressing the underlying cause.

Pelvic inflammatory disease (PID):

PID is an infection of the female reproductive organs, typically caused by sexually transmitted bacteria. It can lead to inflammation, scarring, and damage to the fallopian tubes, uterus, and ovaries. Symptoms may include pelvic pain, abnormal vaginal discharge, painful urination, and fever. Prompt treatment with antibiotics is essential to prevent complications and preserve fertility.

Premenstrual breast tenderness:

Premenstrual breast tenderness refers to breast discomfort, sensitivity, or pain that occurs in the days leading up to menstruation. It is influenced by hormonal changes, specifically fluctuations in estrogen and progesterone levels. Supportive bras, over-the-counter pain relievers, dietary changes, and hormonal therapies can help alleviate the symptoms.

Ovarian Hyper-stimulation Syndrome (OHSS):

OHSS can occur as a result of fertility treatments, particularly in vitro fertilization (IVF). It is characterized by an excessive response of the ovaries to fertility medications, leading to enlarged ovaries, fluid accumulation in the abdomen, and potentially severe complications. Symptoms may include abdominal bloating, nausea, vomiting, and shortness of breath. Close monitoring and medical management are necessary to prevent and treat OHSS.

Uterine bleeding:

Uterine bleeding refers to abnormal bleeding from the uterus, which can occur due to various reasons, including hormonal imbalances, uterine fibroids, polyps, certain medications, or underlying medical conditions. Treatment depends on the cause and may involve hormonal therapies, medication to control bleeding, or surgical interventions.

Vaginal itching and discharge:

Vaginal itching and discharge can be caused by various factors, such as yeast infections, bacterial vaginosis, sexually transmitted infections (STIs), or allergic reactions. Symptoms may include itching, irritation, abnormal discharge, and discomfort. Treatment options range from anti-fungal or antibiotic medications to manage specific infections to lifestyle changes and topical treatments to alleviate symptoms.

Menopause:

Menopause refers to the natural transition in a woman's life when she stops having menstrual periods and is no longer fertile. It is typically a gradual process due to aging and hormonal changes, particularly a decline in estrogen levels. Symptoms may include hot flashes, night sweats, mood changes, vaginal dryness, and sleep disturbances. Hormone therapy, lifestyle adjustments, and symptom management can help women navigate through the menopausal transition.

Breastfeeding issues:

Breastfeeding issues can encompass various challenges that women may experience while nursing their infants. These can include sore nipples, engorgement, low milk supply, mastitis (breast infection), or difficulties with latching or feeding. Support from lactation consultants, proper positioning and latch techniques, managing milk supply, and addressing any underlying issues can help overcome breastfeeding challenges and promote successful breastfeeding.

These are some of these disorders with homeopathic suggestions for the conditions. Once again, this is not to be taken as medical advice in anyway. This is for entertainment purposes only. If you are experiencing any of these medical challenges, please contact a licensed healthcare practitioner.

Menstrual Disorders:

- Pulsatilla: Used for irregular menstrual cycles, late or scanty periods, and mood swings. It may be suitable for individuals who are weepy, clingy, and desire comfort.

- Sepia: Used for heavy or prolonged periods, irritability, fatigue, and indifference toward loved ones. It may be suitable for women who experience hormonal imbalances and mood swings.

- Lachesis: Used for intense menstrual pain, especially on the left side. It may be suitable for women who experience hot flashes, jealousy, and a talkative nature.

Polycystic Ovary Syndrome (PCOS):

- Thuja occidentalis: Used for hormonal imbalances, acne, excess hair growth (hirsutism), and irregular periods. It may suit chilly individuals who tend to develop warts and crave sweets.

- Cyclamen europaeum: Used for irregular periods, PCOS-related symptoms, and mood swings. It may be suitable for women who experience depression, headaches, and dizziness with menstrual irregularities.

- Apis mellifica: Used for ovarian cysts, associated pain, and swelling. It may suit individuals who experience stinging pain and swelling and feel better with cold applications.

Endometriosis:

- Belladonna: Used for severe menstrual cramps, intense pelvic pain, and inflammation. It may be suitable for individuals who have sudden, throbbing pains that are worse with touch or jarring movements.

- Calcarea carbonica: Used for endometriosis-related pelvic pain, heavy bleeding, and fatigue. It may be suitable for individuals who experience prolonged, excessive, and clotted bleeding along with chilliness and weight gain.

- Colocynthis: Used for intense abdominal pain associated with endometriosis, particularly when it feels better by bending double or applying pressure. It may be suitable for individuals who experience cutting colicky pains.

Fibroids:

- Thlaspi bursa-pastoris: Used for heavy bleeding, prolonged periods, and uterine fibroids. It may be suitable for individuals who experience dark, clotted bleeding that is worse with movement and accompanied by fatigue.

- Ustilago maydis: Used for large fibroids, irregular bleeding, and uterine tumors. It may be suitable for individuals who experience profuse, prolonged, and painless bleeding with dark clots.

- Aurum muriaticum natronatum: Used for fibroids accompanied by depression, anxiety, and hopelessness. It may be suitable for individuals who experience heaviness and pressure in the pelvic region.

Vaginal Infections:

- Candida albicans: Used for yeast infections, including symptoms such as itching, burning, and thick discharge. It may be suitable for individuals who experience intense itching and release that is white and cottage cheese-like.

- Borax: Used for vaginal infections with white, watery discharge and increased sensitivity to touch. It may be suitable for individuals who experience a sensation as if warm water is flowing through the vagina.

- Pulsatilla: Used for vaginal infections with thick, yellowish-green discharge and a tendency to feel better in open air. It may be suitable for individuals who experience changeable symptoms and clinginess.

Pelvic Inflammatory Disease (PID):

- Sepia: Used for PID with pelvic pain, vaginal discharge, and hormonal imbalances. It may be suitable for individuals who experience a dragging sensation in the pelvis and have a general feeling of weariness.

- Belladonna: Used for acute, severe cases of PID with intense pelvic pain, fever, and redness. It may be suitable for individuals who experience sudden throbbing pains and have a flushed face.

- Apis mellifica: Used for PID with burning, stinging pain in the pelvis, and swelling. It may be suitable for individuals who experience sharp, severe pains that worsen with touch and are improved by cold applications.

Cervical Cancer:

- Carcinosinum: Used for constitutional support and as an adjunct to conventional treatment for cervical cancer. It may be suitable for individuals who require individualized treatment based on their unique symptoms and characteristics.

- Thuja occidentalis: Used for cervical dysplasia and adjunct to conventional treatment. It may be suitable for individuals who experience warts or other abnormal growths.

Pelvic Organ Prolapse:

- Sepia: Used for pelvic organ prolapse with a sensation of heaviness and bearing down in the pelvis. It may be suitable for individuals who experience worsening symptoms with standing and feel better with rest.

- Bellis perennis: Used for pelvic organ prolapse with bruised and sore sensations. It may be suitable for individuals who experience pain and soreness in the pelvic region after childbirth or surgery.

- Staphysagria: Used for pelvic organ prolapse following childbirth or sexual trauma. It may be suitable for individuals who experience a sensation of weakness and rawness in the pelvic area.

Sexual Dysfunction:

- Lycopodium clavatum: Used for low libido, erectile dysfunction, and performance anxiety. It may be suitable for individuals who experience a lack of self-confidence, digestive issues, and bloating.

- Argentum nitricum: Used for performance anxiety, premature ejaculation, and fear of sexual intimacy. It may be suitable for individuals who experience apprehension and nervousness before sexual encounters.

- Phosphoric acid: Used for sexual exhaustion, loss of libido, and physical weakness. It may suit individuals who experience fatigue, indifference, and emotional exhaustion.

Urinary Incontinence:

- Causticum: Used for stress urinary incontinence, especially coughing or sneezing. It may be suitable for individuals who experience urine leakage due to weakened bladder control.

Vulvodynia:

Kreosotum: Used for vulvodynia with burning, itching, and soreness in the vulvar region. It may be suitable for individuals who experience increased sensitivity to touch and heat.

Staphysagria: Used for vulvodynia related to past trauma or surgery. It may be suitable for individuals who experience a sensation of rawness as if the area has been injured or cut.

Graphites: Used for vulvodynia with rawness, itching, and cracks in the skin. It may suit individuals who experience thick, sticky discharge and constipation.

Pelvic Pain:

Bellis perennis: Used for pelvic pain, especially after childbirth or surgery. It may suit individuals who experience soreness, bruised sensations, and difficulty walking.

Magnesia phosphorica: Used for sharp, shooting pelvic pain relieved by warmth and pressure. It may be suitable for individuals who experience cramping pain and spasms.

Chamomilla: Used for pelvic pain with extreme sensitivity, irritability, and restlessness. It may be suitable for individuals who experience unbearable pain relieved by being carried or rocked.

Uterine Fibroids:

Thlaspi bursa-pastoris: Used for uterine fibroids with heavy bleeding and prolonged periods. It may be suitable for individuals who experience dark, clotted bleeding and feel weak and tired.

Sabina: Used for uterine fibroids with heavy, bright red bleeding and pain that extends to the back. It may be suitable for individuals who experience pain worse from motion and feel better with rest.

Silicea: Used for uterine fibroids with a sensation of pressure and hardness in the abdomen. It may be suitable for individuals who experience easy fatigue, lack of stamina, and sensitivity to cold.

Hormonal Acne:

Natrum muriaticum: Used for hormonal acne with oily skin, especially on the forehead and nose. It may be suitable for individuals who experience acne worsened by stress and feel better in the open air.

Pulsatilla: Used for hormonal acne with red, inflamed eruptions and a tendency to change locations. It may be suitable for individuals who experience acne associated with menstrual irregularities and weepiness.

Sulfur: Used for acne with deep-seated, itchy eruptions and a tendency to worsen with heat. It may suit individuals who experience acne aggravated by washing and improved by dry, warm conditions.

Premenstrual Syndrome (PMS):

Lycopodium clavatum: Used for PMS with bloating, irritability, and sugar cravings. It may be suitable for individuals who experience digestive issues, lack of self-confidence, and mood swings.

Sepia: Used for PMS with mood swings, fatigue, and a sense of indifference. It may be suitable for individuals who feel overwhelmed, irritable, and experience hormonal imbalances.

Nux vomica: Used for PMS with irritability, anger, and digestive issues. It may be suitable for individuals who experience intense cravings, sensitivity to noise, and sleep disturbances.

Ovarian Dysfunction:

Pulsatilla: Used for ovarian dysfunction with irregular or absent periods. It may be suitable for individuals who experience weepiness, clinginess, and a desire for consolation.

Sepia: Used for hormonal imbalances and ovarian dysfunction with a sense of indifference, fatigue, and low libido. It may suit individuals who feel better with vigorous exercise and worse from hormonal changes.

Lilium tigrinum: Used for ovarian dysfunction with depression, anxiety, and irritability. It may be suitable for individuals who experience a sensation of weight or pressure in the pelvis.

Uterine Prolapse:

Sepia: Hypothetically used for uterine prolapse with a heavy, sagging sensation in the pelvis. It may suit individuals who experience bladder weakness, irritability, and exhaustion.

• Bellis perennis: Hypothetically used for uterine prolapse with soreness and bruised feeling in the pelvis. It may be suitable for individuals who experience discomfort after childbirth or injury.

• Murex purpurea: Hypothetically used for uterine prolapse with a bearing down sensation and intense sexual desire. It may be suitable for individuals who experience pain in the pelvis and sensitivity of the vaginal area.

Premenstrual Dysphoric Disorder (PMDD):

• Ignatia amara: Hypothetically used for PMDD with mood swings, weepiness, and emotional sensitivity. It may be suitable for individuals who experience a sense of grief, changeable moods, and sighing.

• Natrum muriaticum: Hypothetically used for PMDD with depression, withdrawal, and salt cravings. It may be suitable for individuals who experience sadness self-isolation and feel worse with consolation.

• Aurum metallicum: Hypothetically used for PMDD with intense sadness, feelings of worthlessness, and self-destructive thoughts. It may be suitable for individuals who experience a sense of hopelessness and a desire to escape.

Cervicitis:

• Sepia: Hypothetically used for cervicitis with vaginal discharge, irritation, and a dragging sensation in the pelvis. It may be suitable for individuals who experience a sense of indifference, fatigue, and hormonal imbalances.

• Kreosotum: Hypothetically used for cervicitis with corrosive, offensive discharge, and burning sensations. It may be suitable for individuals who experience increased sensitivity to touch and tend to feel worse at night.

• Mercurius corrosivus: Hypothetically used for cervicitis with intense burning, stinging pains, and pus-like discharge. It may be suitable for individuals who experience increased salivation and sweating.

Amenorrhea (Absent Menstruation):

• Pulsatilla: Hypothetically used for amenorrhea with irregular or absent periods due to hormonal imbalances. It may be suitable for individuals who experience weepiness, mood swings, and a desire for consolation.

• Natrum muriaticum: Hypothetically used for amenorrhea associated with grief, sadness, and a tendency to isolate oneself. It may suit individuals who feel worse from consolation and strongly need privacy.

• Cyclamen europaeum: Hypothetically used for amenorrhea with irregular periods and hormonal imbalances. It may be suitable for individuals who experience headaches, dizziness, and mood swings with menstrual irregularities.

Vaginismus:

• Lycopodium clavatum: Hypothetically used for vaginismus with involuntary contraction of the vaginal muscles. It may be suitable for individuals who experience anxiety, performance issues, and digestive issues.

• Belladonna: Hypothetically used for vaginismus with intense pain, redness, and sensitivity in the vaginal area. It may be suitable for individuals who experience sudden throbbing pains and have a flushed face.

• Staphysagria: Hypothetically used for vaginismus related to past trauma or sexual abuse. It may be suitable for individuals who experience a sensation of rawness as if the area has been injured or violated.

Vaginal Dryness:

• Sepia: Hypothetically used for vaginal dryness with a sense of indifference, fatigue, and low libido. It may be suitable for individuals who experience dryness along with hormonal imbalances and mood swings.

• Lycopodium clavatum: Hypothetically used for vaginal dryness with itching and burning. It may be suitable for individuals who experience dryness in the vagina, as well as other dry areas like the skin and mucous membranes.

• Natrum muriaticum: Hypothetically used for vaginal dryness associated with grief, sadness, and a tendency to isolate oneself. It may suit individuals who feel worse from consolation and strongly need privacy.

Pelvic Inflammatory Disease (PID):

• Kreosotum: Hypothetically used for PID with offensive vaginal discharge and burning sensations. It may be suitable for individuals who experience increased sensitivity to touch and tenderness in the pelvic region.

• Merc solubilis: Hypothetically used for PID with copious, yellow-green discharge and burning pains. It may suit individuals who experience increased salivation, bad breath, and sweating.

• Hepar sulphuris calcareum: Hypothetically used for PID with sharp, splinter-like pains and foul-smelling discharge. It may be suitable for individuals who feel extremely sensitive to touch and are prone to abscess formation.

Premenstrual Breast Tenderness:

• Conium maculatum: Hypothetically used for breast tenderness before periods, especially when nodules are present. It may be suitable for individuals who experience swollen, hard breasts that are sensitive to touch.

• Belladonna: Hypothetically used for intense breast pain and inflammation before periods. It may be suitable for individuals who experience throbbing pain, redness, and sensitivity in the breasts.

- Bryonia alba: Hypothetically used for breast tenderness worsened by motion and touch. It may be suitable for individuals who experience stitching pain in the breasts and feel relief from firm pressure.

Ovarian Hyper-stimulation Syndrome (OHSS):

- Apis mellifica: Hypothetically used for OHSS with bloating, abdominal discomfort, and fluid retention. It may suit individuals who experience swollen, tender ovaries and feel relief with excellent applications.

- Colchicum: Hypothetically used for OHSS with nausea, vomiting, and abdominal pain. It may be suitable for individuals who experience aversion to food, weakness, and excessive salivation.

- Veratrum album: Hypothetically used for OHSS with profuse diarrhea, cold sweats, and weakness. It may suit individuals who experience intense thirst, coldness, and faintness.

Uterine Bleeding:

- Trillium pendulum: Hypothetically used for uterine bleeding with bright red blood and excessive flow. It may be suitable for individuals who experience a sensation of weight and dragging in the pelvis.

- Sabina: Hypothetically used for uterine bleeding with bright red blood that is accompanied by severe pain. It may be suitable for individuals who experience pain that extends to the back and feel worse from motion.

- China officinalis: Hypothetically used for uterine bleeding with weakness, fatigue, and pale complexion. It may be suitable for individuals who experience profuse bleeding with a sensation of emptiness.

Ovarian Cancer:

- Carcinosinum: Hypothetically used for constitutional support and as an adjunct to conventional treatment for ovarian cancer. It may be suitable for individuals who require individualized treatment based on their unique symptoms and characteristics.

- Conium maculatum: Hypothetically used for ovarian cancer with challenging nodular tumors and swelling. It may be suitable for individuals who experience weakness, vertigo, and a tendency to sweat easily.

- Lachesis: Hypothetically used for ovarian cancer with left-sided symptoms and intense pain. It may be suitable for individuals who experience hot flashes, jealousy, and a talkative nature.

Ovarian Hyper-stimulation Syndrome (OHSS):

- Apis mellifica: Hypothetically used for OHSS with bloating, abdominal discomfort, and fluid retention. It may suit individuals who experience swollen, tender ovaries and feel relief with excellent applications.

- Colchicum: Hypothetically used for OHSS with nausea, vomiting, and abdominal pain. It may be suitable for individuals who experience aversion to food, weakness, and excessive salivation.

- Veratrum album: Hypothetically used for OHSS with profuse diarrhea, cold sweats, and weakness. It may suit individuals who experience intense thirst, coldness, and faintness.

Uterine Bleeding:

- Trillium pendulum: Hypothetically used for uterine bleeding with bright red blood and excessive flow. It may be suitable for individuals who experience a sensation of weight and dragging in the pelvis.

- Sabina: Hypothetically used for uterine bleeding with bright red blood that is accompanied by severe pain. It may be suitable for individuals who experience pain that extends to the back and feel worse from motion.

- China officinalis: Hypothetically used for uterine bleeding with weakness, fatigue, and pale complexion. It may be suitable for individuals who experience profuse bleeding with a sensation of emptiness.

Vaginal Itching and Discharge:

- Sepia: Hypothetically used for vaginal itching and discharge with a dragging sensation in the pelvis. It may be suitable for individuals who experience a sense of indifference, fatigue, and hormonal imbalances.

- Kreosotum: Hypothetically used for vaginal itching and discharge with burning sensations. It may be suitable for individuals who experience increased sensitivity to touch and tenderness in the vaginal area.

- Borax: Hypothetically used for vaginal itching and discharge worsened by touch and triggered by anxiety. It may be suitable for individuals who experience a sensation as if warm water is flowing through the vagina.

Vaginal Yeast Infection:

- Candida albicans: Hypothetically used for vaginal yeast infection with itching, burning, and thick discharge. It may be suitable for individuals who experience intense itching and release that is white and cottage cheese-like.

- Borax: Hypothetically used for vaginal yeast infection with white, watery discharge and increased sensitivity to touch. It may be suitable for individuals who experience a sensation as if warm water is flowing through the vagina.

- Pulsatilla: Hypothetically used for vaginal yeast infection with thick, yellowish-green discharge and a tendency to feel better in open air. It may be suitable for individuals who experience changeable symptoms and clinginess.

Menopausal Symptoms:

- Lachesis: Hypothetically used for hot flashes, mood swings, and other menopausal symptoms. It may be suitable for individuals who experience intense heat vibrations and are talkative.

- Sepia: Hypothetically used for hormonal imbalances, vaginal dryness, low libido, and mood swings during menopause. It may be suitable for individuals who feel overwhelmed irritable, and experience a sense of indifference toward loved ones.

- Sanguinaria canadensis: Hypothetically used for hot flashes, headaches, and migraines during menopause. It may be suitable for individuals who experience flushing of the face, heat, and pulsating headaches.

Breastfeeding Issues:

- Ricinus communis: Hypothetically used for insufficient milk supply and cracked or sore nipples. It may be suitable for individuals who experience dryness and burning sensations.

- Bryonia alba: Hypothetically used for painful and swollen breasts during breastfeeding. It may be suitable for individuals who experience stitching pain in the breasts and feel relief from firm pressure.

- Urtica urens: Hypothetically used for low milk supply and stinging or burning breast pains. It may be suitable for individuals who experience a sensation of heat and increased sensitivity.

The best attributes of men: in praise of manhood

Confidence is a hallmark of manhood, a quiet certainty in one's abilities and decisions that often leads to respect from peers and confidence in oneself. It's not about arrogance but rather a steady, self-assured nature that helps a man navigate life's challenges. This confidence allows a man to stand up for his beliefs, take on responsibilities, and be a pillar of strength for those around him. It can be seen in the way he carries himself, the way he speaks, and the decisions he makes - each reflecting a self-reliance that is both admirable and inspiring.

Leadership is often a role that falls naturally to men, derived from societal expectations and personal inclination. A great leader can inspire, guide, and support others. Leadership in men is not just about being in charge but about taking accountability, encouraging growth in others, and setting a positive example. It's about vision, decision-making, and the capacity to drive a team towards a common goal while respecting and valuing the contributions of each member.

Resilience in the face of adversity is another trait often associated with manhood. This resilience is the inner strength that allows a man to rebound from failure or hardship without losing his heart. It is about facing challenges head-on and emerging on the other side stronger for having gone through them. This quality is essential as it means a man does not shy away from difficult situations but learns from them, demonstrating a robustness of character that helps him persevere.

Compassion may not be the first quality attributed to men, but it is undeniably an outstanding characteristic. Compassion is the empathy and understanding that a man shows towards others. It's a nurturing kind of strength, a willingness to put oneself in another's shoes and act with kindness. A compassionate man builds deep connections with others and creates a sense of trust and safety for those in his life.

Integrity is the moral compass that guides a man through life. It's about honesty, fairness, and consistency in one's beliefs and actions. A man with integrity will stand by his principles even when it is not convenient or advantageous. This adherence to a personal code of ethics earns him the respect of others and a sense of self-respect that is irreplaceable.

Responsibility is often associated with manhood, encompassing both personal duties and responsibilities to others. A responsible man cares for his needs and looks after those dependent on him. He understands the importance of his roles in the family, workplace, and society, and he strives to fulfill his obligations to the best of his ability.

Intellectual curiosity is a characteristic that drives a man to explore, question, and understand the world around him. An intellectually curious man will always be learning, seeking to expand his knowledge and challenge his perspectives. This love for learning contributes to a well-rounded and insightful character.

Humor is a quality that adds brightness to a man's personality. A good sense of humor can diffuse tension, unite people, and relieve difficult situations. A man who can laugh at himself and find joy in life's absurdities can often navigate life with a lighter heart and a more positive outlook.

Commitment is a deep-seated characteristic that shows a man's reliability and dedication. Whether it is a commitment to a relationship, a cause, or a goal, this trait demonstrates a man's ability to be steadfast and unwavering in his pursuits. It's about a long-term dedication that outlasts fleeting desires and challenges.

Protectiveness in a man can be a profound trait. It is a characteristic that manifests not in a desire to control but in the impulse to ensure the safety and well-being of loved ones. A protective man provides security to those in his care, offering support and defense against physical and emotional harm.

Creativity is not confined by gender and is an excellent attribute for a man. Creativity fuels innovation and problem-solving. A creative man approaches challenges uniquely and contributes original ideas and solutions personally and professionally.

Courage is often associated with manhood; it's the ability to face fear, uncertainty, and intimidation without being deterred. A courageous man does not lack fear, but he confronts it, whether in the form of physical challenges, standing up for his convictions, or making difficult decisions.

Patience is a virtue that is valuable for a man to have. It's the ability to endure difficult circumstances with perseverance and poise. A patient man can handle stress and frustration without becoming overwhelmed or acting impulsively, which allows for thoughtful decision-making and a calm presence for those around him.

Generosity in a man enriches not only the lives of others but also his own life. It is not just about giving materially but also about being generous with time, attention, and spirit. A helpful man shares what he has, whether it is knowledge, resources, or a helping hand, and does so without expecting anything in return.

Discipline is a characteristic that empowers a man to achieve his goals. It is the practice of training oneself to be consistent, focused, and in control of one's appetites and behaviors. A disciplined man can set goals and work diligently, maintaining his direction despite distractions or temptations.

Adaptability is a quality that is particularly valuable in the fast-paced, ever-changing modern world. An adaptable man can navigate changes in circumstances, roles, or environments with ease and grace. This flexibility of mind and approach allows him to overcome obstacles and adjust his strategies as necessary.

Loyalty is a characteristic that fosters deep and lasting relationships. A loyal man stands by his friends, family, and partners, offering them support and fidelity. This loyalty builds strong bonds and a reputation for reliability and trustworthiness.

Ambition in a man is the driving force behind personal and professional growth. An ambitious man sets his sights on his goals and works tirelessly to achieve them. This ambition is not selfish; instead, it can lead to advancements and contributions that benefit society.

Practicality is a quality that serves a man well in everyday life. A practical man can sensibly approach problems and situations, finding workable solutions and making decisions based on realistic considerations.

Empathy is the capacity to understand and share the feelings of another, and in a man, it can break down barriers and foster connections. An empathetic man can offer support that is both genuine and profound, providing comfort and understanding in times of need.

Here is a list of health topics that commonly affect men:

Disclaimer: This information is purely for entertainment purposes only. The following list of homeopathic remedies is intended for entertainment and should not be considered medical advice. It is essential to consult a certified and licensed healthcare practitioner before proceeding with any of the information provided below, especially if you are experiencing any of the mentioned symptoms or health conditions.

Premature Ejaculation:

Premature ejaculation occurs when ejaculation happens too quickly during sexual activity, leading to unsatisfactory sexual experiences. It is one of the most common sexual problems in men. Behavioral techniques, topical numbing agents, and medication can be used for management.

Prostate Enlargement (Benign Prostatic Hyperplasia - BPH):

Benign prostatic hyperplasia (BPH) is a non-cancerous prostate gland enlargement common in aging men. It can cause urinary difficulties, such as frequent urination, weak urine stream, or difficulty starting and stopping urination. Treatment options include medication, minimally invasive procedures, and surgery.

Prostate Cancer:

Prostate cancer is the development of cancerous cells in the prostate gland. It is the second most common cancer in men worldwide. Treatment options depend on the stage and aggressiveness of the cancer and may include surgery, radiation therapy, hormone therapy, chemotherapy, and immunotherapy.

Testicular Cancer:

Testicular cancer is the growth of cancerous cells in the testicles. It most commonly affects younger men. Treatment involves surgical removal of the affected testicle, followed by further treatment like radiation therapy or chemotherapy if necessary.

Male Infertility:

Male infertility refers to the inability to conceive a child due to factors affecting sperm production, motility, or function. Causes can include hormonal imbalances, testicular injuries, infections, or genetic factors. Treatment options depend on the underlying cause and may involve medication, surgery, or assisted reproductive technologies like in vitro fertilization (IVF).

Prostatitis:

Prostatitis is the inflammation of the prostate gland, leading to urinary issues and pelvic pain. It can be acute or chronic, and treatment depends on the type and underlying cause. Antibiotics, alpha-blockers, and pain relievers are common treatments.

Andropause (Male Menopause):

Andropause refers to an age-related decline in testosterone levels, leading to various symptoms like fatigue, reduced muscle mass, mood changes, and decreased sexual desire. Hormone replacement therapy may be considered for symptom management.

Low Testosterone (Hypogonadism):

Hypogonadism is the insufficient production of testosterone. Medical conditions, injuries, or genetic factors can cause it. Treatment options include testosterone replacement therapy in the form of gels, patches, injections, or pellets.

Male Pattern Baldness (Androgenetic Alopecia):

Male pattern baldness is a genetic condition causing hair loss, typically affecting the hairline and crown of the head. Treatment options include medications like minoxidil and finasteride, hair transplant surgery, and low-level laser therapy.

Male Breast Enlargement (Gynecomastia):

Gynecomastia is the enlargement of breast tissue in males, often due to hormonal imbalances. In most cases, gynecomastia resolves on its own. Surgery may be considered for severe or persistent cases.

Depression:

Depression is a mood disorder characterized by persistent sadness, loss of interest, changes in sleep and appetite, and feelings of hopelessness. It can affect men of all ages, and treatment may involve therapy, medication, or a combination of both.

Anxiety Disorders:

Anxiety disorders involve excessive worry, fear, and nervousness that can significantly impact daily life. Treatment options include therapy, medication, and stress-reducing techniques.

Cardiovascular Diseases:

Cardiovascular diseases encompass a group of conditions affecting the heart and blood vessels. Common cardiovascular conditions in men include coronary artery disease, heart attacks, and strokes. Lifestyle changes, medication, and medical procedures manage these conditions.

Hypertension (High Blood Pressure):

Hypertension is persistently elevated blood pressure, a significant risk factor for heart disease and stroke. Lifestyle modifications and medication are commonly used to manage hypertension.

Diabetes:

Diabetes is a chronic condition characterized by high blood sugar levels. It can lead to various complications if not managed well. Treatment involves blood sugar monitoring, lifestyle changes, and medication.

Chronic Obstructive Pulmonary Disease (COPD):

COPD includes chronic bronchitis and emphysema, progressive lung diseases often caused by smoking. Smoking cessation, inhalers, and oxygen therapy are used in COPD management.

Sleep Apnea:

Sleep apnea is a sleep disorder where breathing repeatedly stops and starts during sleep, leading to poor sleep quality and daytime fatigue. Continuous positive airway pressure (CPAP) therapy and lifestyle changes are commonly used treatments.

Alcohol Use Disorder:

Alcohol use disorder involves a pattern of drinking that leads to significant distress or impairment in daily life. Treatment may include counseling, support groups, and medication.

Drug Abuse and Addiction:

Drug abuse and addiction refer to the misuse of drugs, leading to physical and psychological dependence. Treatment may involve detoxification, counseling, and support groups.

Obesity:

Obesity is excessive body weight, increasing the risk of various health conditions. Lifestyle changes, diet, and exercise are essential components of obesity management.

Osteoporosis:

Osteoporosis is characterized by weakened bones, increasing the risk of fractures. Adequate calcium and vitamin D intake, weight-bearing exercises, and medication are used in osteoporosis management.

Chronic Kidney Disease:

Chronic kidney disease is long-term kidney damage, reducing the ability to filter waste and fluids from the blood. Management involves lifestyle changes, medication, and dialysis or kidney transplants in severe cases.

Anemia:

Anemia is a deficiency in red blood cells or hemoglobin, leading to fatigue and weakness. Treatment may involve iron supplementation and addressing the underlying cause.

Inguinal Hernia:

An inguinal hernia occurs when a part of the intestine or abdominal tissue protrudes through a weakened area in the abdominal wall, usually near the groin. It can cause a visible bulge and discomfort, especially when lifting or straining. Surgery is the most common treatment for inguinal hernias to repair the weakened abdominal wall and return the herniated tissue to its proper position.

Varicocele:

Varicoceles are enlarged veins in the scrotum, similar to varicose veins in the legs. They can affect sperm production and male fertility by increasing testicular temperature and impairing blood flow. Treatment options depend on the severity of symptoms and fertility concerns and may include surgical repair or embolization to redirect blood flow away from the affected veins.

Obstructive Sleep Apnea:

Obstructive sleep apnea is a sleep disorder where the airway becomes blocked or collapses during sleep, leading to interrupted breathing and reduced oxygen intake. This can result in fragmented sleep and excessive daytime sleepiness. Continuous positive airway pressure (CPAP) therapy is the most common treatment, using a machine to deliver air pressure through a mask to keep the airway open.

Testicular Torsion:

Testicular torsion is a medical emergency where the spermatic cord twists, cutting off blood flow to the testicle. It presents with sudden and severe testicular pain, swelling, and possible nausea. Immediate surgical intervention is necessary to untwist the cord and restore blood flow to prevent permanent damage to the testicle.

Epididymitis:

Epididymitis is the inflammation of the epididymis, the tube at the back of the testicles that stores and carries sperm. It can be caused by infections, sexually transmitted diseases, or urinary tract infections. Symptoms include pain, swelling, and discomfort in the scrotum. Additional symptoms may include redness, warmth, tenderness, and a lump in the affected area. Prompt medical attention is crucial to determine the underlying cause and provide appropriate treatment, including antibiotics, pain relief, and rest to alleviate symptoms and prevent complications.

Balanitis:

Balanitis is the inflammation of the glans penis, typically caused by an infection or poor hygiene. Symptoms include redness, soreness, itching, and discharge. Pain or discomfort during urination, swelling, an unpleasant odor, and difficulty retracting the foreskin may also be experienced. Proper hygiene practices, including gentle cleaning of the penis and avoiding irritants, can help prevent balanitis. Treatment may include topical or oral medications to address infections, along with supportive measures to alleviate symptoms and promote healing.

Fungal Infections (e.g., jock itch):

Fungal infections, such as jock itch, are caused by fungal overgrowth in warm and moist areas of the body, commonly affecting the groin area. These infections result in redness, itching, and a rash in the affected area. Other symptoms may include a burning sensation, flaking or peeling skin, a distinctive ring-shaped pattern of inflammation, and the presence of blisters or ulcers. Proper hygiene, keeping the area dry, and antifungal treatments are typically used to manage fungal infections effectively.

Urinary Tract Infections (UTIs):

Urinary tract infections (UTIs) affect the urinary system, including the bladder and urethra. They can cause painful urination, frequent urges to urinate, and a feeling of incomplete bladder emptying. UTIs can be caused by bacteria entering the urinary tract. Treatment involves antibiotics to clear the infection and prevent complications.

Inguinal Groin Pain:

Inguinal groin pain is discomfort or pain in the region, often caused by muscle strains, hernias, or referred pain from other areas. Treatment depends on the underlying cause and may include rest, physical therapy, or surgery for hernias.

Sports Injuries:

Various sports injuries can affect men, including strains, sprains, fractures, and joint injuries. Proper warm-up, stretching, and conditioning can help prevent sports-related injuries. Treatment varies depending on the type and severity of the injury and may include rest, physical therapy, or surgical intervention.

Hypertrophic Cardiomyopathy:

Hypertrophic cardiomyopathy is a genetic heart condition where the heart muscle thickens, potentially leading to heart failure. Treatment focuses on managing symptoms reducing the risk of complications, and may include medications, lifestyle changes, and, in severe cases, surgical interventions.

Colon Cancer:

Colon cancer is the development of cancerous cells in the colon or rectum. Regular screening and early detection are essential for successful treatment. Treatment options include surgery, radiation therapy, chemotherapy, and targeted therapy, depending on the stage and extent of the cancer.

Anxiety Disorders:

Anxiety disorders involve excessive worry, fear, and nervousness that can significantly impact daily life. Treatment options include therapy, medication, and stress-reducing techniques.

Rheumatoid Arthritis:

Rheumatoid arthritis is an autoimmune disease-causing joint pain, stiffness, and inflammation. Early diagnosis and treatment are crucial to manage symptoms and prevent joint damage. Treatments may include medications, physical therapy, and lifestyle changes.

Chronic Fatigue Syndrome (CFS):

Chronic fatigue syndrome is characterized by severe fatigue that persists for an extended period, negatively affecting daily functioning. There is no specific cure for CFS, and treatment focuses on symptom management, including lifestyle changes, rest, and pacing activities.

Psoriasis:

Psoriasis is a chronic skin condition characterized by red, scaly patches of skin. Treatment options include topical creams, phototherapy, and systemic medications.

Azoospermia (No Sperm in Semen):

Azoospermia refers to a condition where sperm are absent in the semen. It can result from hormonal imbalances, genetic factors, obstruction in the reproductive tract, or testicular abnormalities, leading to male infertility.

Vaginal Discharge (in Male):

Vaginal discharge in males refers to the abnormal release of fluid from the urethra. It may be caused by infections, inflammation of the urethra, or sexually transmitted diseases.

Breast Cancer (in Men):

Breast cancer in men is the development of cancerous cells in the breast tissue. It is relatively rare in males but can occur and may present as a lump or swelling in the breast tissue.

Infertility (Male Factor):

Male infertility is the inability to achieve pregnancy due to issues with sperm production, function, or delivery. It can result from hormonal imbalances, genetic factors, infections, or lifestyle choices.

Gynecomastia (Enlarged Male Breasts):

Gynecomastia is the enlargement of male breast tissue, resulting in a swollen appearance. It can occur due to hormonal imbalances, obesity, certain medications, or underlying medical conditions.

Urinary Incontinence:

Urinary incontinence is the involuntary loss of urine, leading to leakage from the bladder. Weak bladder muscles, nerve damage, or an enlarged prostate gland can cause it.

Hemorrhoids (Piles):

Hemorrhoids, also known as piles, are swollen and inflamed veins in the lower rectum and anus. They can cause pain, itching, and bleeding during bowel movements.

Varicose Veins:

Varicose veins are enlarged, swollen, and twisted, usually in the legs. They result from weakened vein walls and malfunctioning valves.

Hair Loss (Male Pattern Baldness):

Male pattern baldness is a common form of hair loss in men characterized by a receding hairline and thinning hair on the crown of the head. Genetic factors and hormonal changes usually cause it.

Gout:

A gout is a form of arthritis characterized by sudden, severe attacks of pain, redness, and tenderness in the joints, commonly affecting the big toe. It is caused by an accumulation of uric acid crystals in the joints.

Liver Cirrhosis:

Liver cirrhosis is a late stage scarring of the liver caused by many forms of liver diseases and conditions, such as hepatitis and chronic alcoholism. It results in impaired liver function and various complications.

Parkinson's Disease:

Parkinson's disease is a progressive nervous system disorder that affects movement, causing tremors, stiffness, and difficulty with walking and coordination. The loss of dopamine-producing brain cells causes it.

Autism Spectrum Disorder (ASD):

Autism spectrum disorder is a developmental disorder that affects communication, behavior, and social interaction. It is a broad range of conditions, and symptoms may vary significantly.

Erectile Dysfunction (ED):

Erectile dysfunction is the inability to achieve or maintain an erection sufficient for sexual activity. It can result from physical or psychological factors, such as vascular issues, hormonal imbalances, or stress.

Benign Prostatic Hyperplasia (BPH):

Benign prostatic hyperplasia is the prostate gland enlargement that commonly occurs with age. It can cause urinary symptoms, such as frequent urination and weak urine flow.

Obsessive-Compulsive Disorder (OCD):

Obsessive-compulsive disorder is a mental health disorder characterized by obsessive thoughts and compulsive behaviors. Individuals may engage in repetitive actions to alleviate anxiety or intrusive thoughts.

Alopecia Areata:

Alopecia areata is an autoimmune condition that causes sudden hair loss in small, round patches on the scalp or other body areas.

Laryngitis:

Laryngitis is larynx inflammation (voice box) that leads to hoarseness or loss of voice. Infections, vocal strain, or irritants can cause it.

Gastritis:

Gastritis is inflammation of the stomach lining, resulting in symptoms such as nausea, indigestion, and abdominal pain.

Sinusitis:

Sinusitis is inflammation of the sinuses, air-filled spaces in the skull. It can cause nasal congestion, facial pain, and headache.

Ear Infections (Otitis Media):

Otitis media is inflammation of the middle ear, often caused by bacterial or viral infections. It can result in ear pain, fluid buildup, and temporary hearing loss.

Nasal Polyps:

Nasal polyps are noncancerous growths that develop in the nose lining or sinuses, leading to nasal congestion and difficulty breathing.

Anemia:

Anemia is when the body lacks enough healthy red blood cells to carry sufficient oxygen to the tissues. It can lead to fatigue, weakness, and pale skin.

Fatty Liver Disease (Non-Alcoholic):

Non-alcoholic fatty liver disease is the accumulation of fat in the liver without alcohol consumption. It can lead to liver inflammation and scarring.

Hypothyroidism:

Hypothyroidism is an under-active thyroid gland, leading to reduced production of thyroid hormones and resulting in symptoms such as fatigue, weight gain, and sensitivity to cold.

Prostate Cancer:

Prostate cancer is the development of cancerous cells in the prostate gland. It is one of the most common cancers in men.

Polycystic Ovary Syndrome (PCOS) in Men (Stein-Leventhal Syndrome):

PCOS in men is a rare condition characterized by hormonal imbalances, which may lead to symptoms such as irregular periods, weight gain, and infertility.

Prostatitis (Chronic Nonbacterial):

Chronic nonbacterial prostatitis is inflammation of the prostate gland without a bacterial infection. It can cause urinary symptoms and discomfort in the pelvic region.

Chlamydia Infection (Genital Chlamydia):

Chlamydia infection is a common sexually transmitted infection caused by the bacterium Chlamydia trachomatis. It can lead to genital and urinary symptoms but often remains asymptomatic.

Erectile Dysfunction (Impotence):

- Agnus castus: This remedy is beneficial for men with low sexual desire, premature ejaculation, and erectile dysfunction resulting from depression, anxiety, or overindulgence in sexual activities.

- Lycopodium clavatum: Used for impotence accompanied by feelings of inadequacy and performance anxiety. Men needing Lycopodium may have difficulty getting an erection, but once achieved, it may be lost during intercourse.

- Selenium metallicum: This remedy is prescribed for erectile dysfunction linked to excessive sexual activity, exhaustion, and weakness.

- Acidum phosphoricum: Men experiencing loss of sexual power due to grief, sadness, or mental exhaustion may benefit from this remedy.

- Aurum metallicum: This remedy is used for impotence in men with feelings of worthlessness, intense stress, and depression.

Premature Ejaculation:

- Staphysagria: This remedy is helpful for men experiencing premature ejaculation with suppressed emotions, especially anger or resentment.

- Graphites: Men needing Graphites may experience premature ejaculation due to anxiety, timidity, and sensitivity.

- Gelsemium sempervirens: Prescribed for men with premature ejaculation due to performance anxiety and fear of public speaking or stage fright.

- Avena sativa: This remedy is helpful for premature ejaculation linked to sexual exhaustion and nervous debility.

- Titanium metallicum: Used for premature ejaculation with excessive sensitivity and irritability.

Inguinal Hernia:

- Nux vomica: This remedy is used for inguinal hernia related to strain, overexertion, or sedentary lifestyle.

- Bryonia alba: Prescribed for inguinal hernia aggravated by movement and relieved by rest.

- Colocynthis: Used for inguinal hernia with cramping and shooting pain.

- Rhus Toxicodendron: This remedy is beneficial for inguinal hernia caused by overexertion and relieved by movement.

- Belladonna: Prescribed for sudden and intense inguinal hernia with redness and heat.

Andropause (Male Menopause):

- Lycopodium clavatum: Used for andropause with physical and mental exhaustion, decreased libido, and performance anxiety.

- Phosphoricum acidum: This remedy is beneficial for andropause with emotional exhaustion, indifference, and apathy.

- Agnus castus: Prescribed for andropause with reduced sexual desire, premature ejaculation, and erectile dysfunction.

- Selenium metallicum: Used for andropause with weakness, fatigue, and sexual debility.

- Acidum phosphoricum: This remedy is helpful for andropause with mental and physical exhaustion, including cases of sexual weakness.

Menopause in Men (Andropause):

- Lycopodium clavatum: Prescribed for andropause with physical and mental exhaustion, decreased libido, and performance anxiety.

- Phosphoricum acidum: Used for andropause with emotional exhaustion, indifference, and apathy.

- Agnus castus: This remedy is beneficial for andropause with reduced sexual desire, premature ejaculation, and erectile dysfunction.

- Selenium metallicum: Used for andropause with weakness, fatigue, and sexual debility.

- Acidum phosphoricum: Prescribed for andropause with mental and physical exhaustion, including cases of sexual weakness.

Oligospermia (Low Sperm Count):

- Agnus castus: Used for oligospermia with reduced sexual desire, premature ejaculation, and erectile dysfunction.

- Lycopodium clavatum: Prescribed for oligospermia accompanied by hormonal imbalances, erectile dysfunction, and premature ejaculation.

- Selenium metallicum: This remedy is helpful for sexual weakness, exhaustion, and oligospermia.

- Acidum phosphoricum: Used for mental and physical exhaustion, including cases of oligospermia.

- Aurum metallicum: Prescribed for depression, anxiety, and oligospermia related to emotional stress.

Azoospermia (No Sperm in Semen):

- Lycopodium clavatum: This remedy is beneficial for azoospermia accompanied by hormonal imbalances, erectile dysfunction, and premature ejaculation.

- Selenium metallicum: Used for sexual weakness, exhaustion, and azoospermia.

- Acidum phosphoricum: Prescribed for mental and physical exhaustion, including cases of azoospermia.

- Aurum metallicum: This remedy is helpful for depression, anxiety, and azoospermia related to emotional stress.

- Conium maculatum: Prescribed for azoospermia when there is swelling, induration, and hardness of glands.

Prostate Enlargement (BPH):

- Sabal serrulata: This remedy is beneficial for prostate enlargement with difficulty in initiating urine flow and frequent urination, especially at night.

- Chimaphila umbellata: Used for prostate enlargement with difficulty in urination and burning pain while passing urine.

- Conium maculatum: Prescribed for prostate enlargement with interrupted and weak urine flow.

- Pulsatilla pratensis: Used for prostate enlargement with a frequent urge to urinate and difficulty in passing urine.

- Thuja occidentalis: This remedy is helpful for prostate enlargement with dribbling of urine and difficulty in emptying the bladder.

Testicular Cancer and Prostate Cancer:

- Conium maculatum: This remedy is indicated for testicular and prostate cancer when there is swelling, induration, and hardness of glands. It may also help with urinary difficulties.

- Carcinosinum: Used for cancer-related symptoms and support in cancer cases.

- Thuja occidentalis: Prescribed for cancer-related symptoms, skin issues, and hormonal imbalances.

- Hydrastis canadensis: Beneficial for cancer symptoms and general immune support.

- Scrophularia nodosa: Used for swollen glands and cancer-related symptoms.

Male Infertility:
- Agnus castus: This remedy is helpful for low libido and sexual weakness in cases of male infertility.
- Lycopodium clavatum: Prescribed for male infertility accompanied by hormonal imbalances, erectile dysfunction, and premature ejaculation.
- Selenium metallicum: Used for sexual weakness, exhaustion, and male infertility.
- Acidum phosphoricum: This remedy is helpful for mental and physical exhaustion, including cases of male infertility.
- Aurum metallicum: Prescribed for depression, anxiety, and male fertility issues related to emotional stress.
Depression and Anxiety Disorders:
- Ignatia amara: Used for individuals experiencing deep grief, sadness, and mood swings. Ignatia is beneficial for emotional sensitivity and suppression of feelings.
- Natrum muriaticum: This remedy is helpful for people who internalize their emotions, especially grief and disappointment. It is used for individuals who may appear reserved or distant but experience deep emotional turmoil.
- Arsenicum album: Prescribed for anxiety and restlessness with fear of death, health concerns, and desire for reassurance and company.
- Pulsatilla pratensis: Used for emotional instability, weepiness, and mood swings, especially during hormonal changes.
- Gelsemium sempervirens: This remedy benefits anxiety and anticipatory fears, especially before important events or performances.
Cardiovascular Diseases:

- Crataegus oxyacantha: Prescribed for heart weakness and cardiovascular conditions, including irregular heartbeat and hypertension.

- Digitalis purpurea: Used for heart issues with weak pulse, irregular heartbeat, and symptoms of heart failure.

- Baryta carbonica: This remedy is helpful for high blood pressure in elderly individuals with a weak and enlarged heart.

- Naja triptans: Beneficial for heart problems, palpitations, and chest pain.

- Aurum metallicum: Prescribed for depression, anxiety, and heart issues related to emotional stress.

Hypertension (High Blood Pressure):

- Baryta muriatic: This remedy is used for high blood pressure in young individuals, primarily due to stress or emotional sensitivity.

- Glonoinum: Prescribed for hypertension with a sudden and severe headache and palpitations.

- Rauwolfia serpentina: Used for hypertension with dizziness, flushing, and pounding in the head.

-

Viscum album: This remedy is helpful for hypertension in elderly individuals with a tendency to faint.

- Syzygium jambolanum: Used for diabetes with excessive thirst, frequent urination, and weakness.

- Uranium nitricum: Prescribed for diabetes with increased appetite, excessive thirst, and emaciation.

- Phosphoricum acidum: This remedy is beneficial for diabetes with physical and mental exhaustion, especially after grief or emotional shock.

- Natrum sulphuricum: Used for diabetes with water retention, bloating, and liver-related symptoms.

- Abroma Augusta: Prescribed for diabetes with increased appetite, weight loss, and weakness.

Chronic Obstructive Pulmonary Disease (COPD):
- Arsenicum album: Used for COPD with anxiety, restlessness, and difficulty breathing, especially at night.
- Antimonium tartaricum: This remedy is helpful for COPD with excessive mucus production, difficulty coughing up phlegm, and rattling in the chest.
- Blatta orientalis: Prescribed for COPD with a cough, difficulty breathing, and constriction in the chest.
- Sambucus nigra: Used for COPD with sudden and severe breathing difficulties, especially in children and infants.
- Lobelia inflata: This remedy is helpful for COPD with shortness of breath and feelings of suffocation.
Sleep Apnea:
- Opium: Used for sleep apnea with heavy snoring and drowsiness during the day.
- Sambucus nigra: Prescribed for sleep apnea in children and infants with difficulty breathing during sleep.
- Chamomilla: This remedy benefits sleep apnea with restlessness, irritability, and difficulty falling asleep.
- Nux vomica: Used for sleep apnea related to digestive issues, alcohol, or caffeine consumption.
- Coffea cruda: This remedy is helpful for sleep apnea with an inability to sleep and an overactive mind.
Varicocele:
- Arnica montana: Prescribed for varicocele with soreness, bruised feeling, and discomfort in the affected area.
- Hamamelis virginiana: Used for varicocele with a sensation of fullness, pain, and tenderness in the scrotum.

- Pulsatilla pratensis: This remedy is helpful for varicocele with swelling, heaviness, and relief from cold applications.

- Lycopodium clavatum: Used for varicocele with right-sided symptoms, swelling, and digestive issues.

- Aurum metallicum: Prescribed for varicocele with depression, anxiety, and emotional stress.

Inguinal Groin Pain:

- Nux vomica: Used for inguinal groin pain related to strain, overexertion, or sedentary lifestyle.

- Bryonia alba: Prescribed for inguinal groin pain aggravated by movement and relieved by rest.

- Colocynthis: This remedy is beneficial for inguinal groin pain with cramping and shooting pain.

- Rhus Toxicodendron: Used for inguinal groin pain caused by overexertion and relieved by movement.

- Belladonna: This remedy is helpful for sudden and intense inguinal groin pain with redness and heat.

Sports Injuries:

- Arnica Montana: Prescribed for sports injuries with bruising, soreness, and trauma to soft tissues.

- Rhus Toxicodendron: Used for sports injuries with stiffness, pain, and aggravation from rest.

- Bryonia alba: This remedy benefits sports injuries with sharp and stitching pain aggravated by movement.

- Ruta graveolens: Used for sports injuries involving tendons, ligaments, and bruised bones.

- Calcarea phosphorica: Prescribed for sports injuries with slow healing, fractures, and bone pain.

Hypertrophic Cardiomyopathy:

- Crataegus oxyacantha: Used for heart weakness and cardiovascular conditions, including hypertrophic cardiomyopathy.

- Digitalis purpurea: This remedy is helpful for hypertrophic cardiomyopathy with irregular heartbeat and palpitations.
- Baryta carbonica: Prescribed for high blood pressure in elderly individuals with a weak and enlarged heart.
- Naja triptans: Beneficial for heart problems, palpitations, and chest pain.
- Aurum metallicum: This remedy is used for depression, anxiety, and heart issues related to emotional stress.

Colon Cancer:
- Conium maculatum: This remedy is indicated for colon cancer when there is swelling, induration, and hardness of glands. It may also help with urinary difficulties.
- Carcinosinum: Used for cancer-related symptoms and support in cancer cases.
- Thuja occidentalis: Prescribed for cancer-related symptoms, skin issues, and hormonal imbalances.
- Hydrastis canadensis: Beneficial for cancer symptoms and general immune support.
- Scrophularia nodosa: Used for swollen glands and cancer-related symptoms.

Bacterial Prostatitis:
- Apis mellifica: Prescribed for bacterial prostatitis with inflammation, burning, and stinging pain during urination.
- Clematis erecta: This remedy is beneficial for prostatitis with a frequent urge to urinate and difficulty passing urine.
- Mercurius corrosives: Used for bacterial prostatitis with intense burning and painful urination.
- Pulsatilla pratensis: Prescribed for prostatitis with a sensation of fullness, heaviness, and discomfort in the pelvis.
- Rhododendron chrysanthum: Beneficial for prostatitis with aching, soreness, and radiating pain in the back and hips.

Epididymitis:

- Apis mellifica: This remedy is used for epididymitis with swelling, redness, and stinging pain in the scrotum.

- Clematis recta: Prescribed for epididymitis with painful swelling and drawing pain in the testicles.

- Mercurius corrosives: Used for epididymitis with intense burning, stitching pain, and difficulty passing urine.

- Pulsatilla pratensis: This remedy is helpful for epididymitis with a sensation of fullness, heaviness, and relief from cold applications.

- Rhododendron chrysanthum: Beneficial for epididymitis with aching, soreness, and drawing pain in the testicles.

Balanitis:

- Calendula officinalis: Prescribed for balanitis with inflammation, redness, and soreness of the glans penis.

- Cantharis vesicatoria: Used for balanitis with burning, smarting pain, and painful urination.

- Graphites: This remedy benefits balanitis with cracked, dry skin and sticky discharge.

- Mezereum: Used for balanitis with itching, burning, and crusty eruptions on the glans penis.

- Sepia officinalis: Prescribed for balanitis with redness, itching, and burning sensations.

Fungal Infections (e.g., jock itch):

- Sulphur: Used for fungal infections with redness, itching, and burning sensations.

- Sepia officinalis: Prescribed for fungal infections with moist, offensive-smelling discharges and itchiness.

- Thuja occidentalis: This remedy is beneficial for fungal infections with warts or growths on the skin.

- Graphites: Used for fungal infections with raw, red, and cracked skin.

- Natrum muriaticum: Prescribed for fungal infections with itching and skin eruptions, worsened by heat.

Urinary Tract Infections (UTIs):

- Cantharis vesicatoria: This remedy is used for UTIs with intense burning pain during urination and a frequent urge to urinate.

- Apis mellifica: Prescribed for UTIs with stinging, smarting pain, and scanty, milky urine.

- Staphysagria: Used for UTIs caused by irritation after sexual intercourse or suppressed emotions.

- Sarsaparilla officinalis: This remedy is beneficial for UTIs with burning pain at the end of urination and kidney colic.

- Pulsatilla pratensis: Prescribed for UTIs with mild, changeable symptoms and a desire for open air.

Hydrocele:

- Apis mellifica: Used for hydrocele with swelling, soreness, and aching pain in the scrotum.

- Arnica montana: Prescribed for hydrocele with soreness, bruised feeling, and discomfort in the affected area.

- Pulsatilla pratensis: This remedy is helpful for hydrocele with swelling, heaviness, and relief from cold applications.

- Rhododendron chrysanthum: Used for hydrocele with aching, soreness, and drawing pain in the testicles.

- Silicea: Prescribed for hydrocele with swelling and hardness in the scrotum.

Breast Cancer (in Men):

- Conium maculatum: Prescribed for breast cancer in men when there is swelling, induration, and hardness of glands.

- Carcinosinum: Used for cancer-related symptoms and support in cancer cases.

- Thuja occidentalis: This remedy benefits cancer-related symptoms, skin issues, and hormonal imbalances.

- Hydrastis canadensis: Used for cancer symptoms and general immune support.

- Scrophularia nodosa: Prescribed for swollen glands and cancer-related symptoms.

Infertility (Male Factor):

- Agnus castus: Used for low libido and sexual weakness in cases of male infertility.

- Lycopodium clavatum: Prescribed for male infertility accompanied by hormonal imbalances, erectile dysfunction, and premature ejaculation.

- Selenium metallicum: This remedy is helpful for sexual weakness, exhaustion, and male infertility.

- Acidum phosphoricum: Used for mental and physical exhaustion, including cases of male infertility.

- Aurum metallicum: Prescribed for depression, anxiety, and male fertility issues related to emotional stress.

Gynecomastia (Enlarged Male Breasts):

- Conium maculatum: This remedy is used for gynecomastia with swollen, painful breasts.

- Thuja occidentalis: Prescribed for gynecomastia with hard, knotty, or nodular growths in the breasts.

- Graphites: Used for gynecomastia with enlarged breasts and dry, cracked skin.

- Rhus Toxicodendron: This remedy benefits gynecomastia

Sepia officinalis: Prescribed for fungal infections with moist, offensive-smelling discharges and itchiness.

- Thuja occidentalis: This remedy is beneficial for fungal infections with warts or growths on the skin.

- Graphites: Used for fungal infections with raw, red, and cracked skin.

- Natrum muriaticum: Prescribed for fungal infections with itching and skin eruptions, worsened by heat.

Urinary Tract Infections (UTIs):

- Cantharis vesicatoria: This remedy is used for UTIs with intense burning pain during urination and a frequent urge to urinate.

- Apis mellifica: Prescribed for UTIs with stinging, smarting pain, and scanty, milky urine.

- Staphysagria: Used for UTIs caused by irritation after sexual intercourse or suppressed emotions.

- Sarsaparilla officinalis: This remedy is beneficial for UTIs with burning pain at the end of urination and kidney colic.

- Pulsatilla pratensis: Prescribed for UTIs with mild, changeable symptoms and a desire for open air.

Inguinal Hernia:

- Nux vomica: This remedy is used for inguinal hernia related to strain, overexertion, or sedentary lifestyle.

- Bryonia alba: Prescribed for inguinal hernia aggravated by movement and relieved by rest.

- Colocynthis: Used for inguinal hernia with cramping and shooting pain.

- Rhus Toxicodendron: This remedy is beneficial for inguinal hernia caused by overexertion and relieved by movement.

- Belladonna: Prescribed for sudden and intense inguinal hernia with redness and heat.

Andropause (Male Menopause):

- Lycopodium clavatum: Used for andropause with physical and mental exhaustion, decreased libido, and performance anxiety.

- Phosphoricum acidum: This remedy is beneficial for andropause with emotional exhaustion, indifference, and apathy.

- Agnus castus: Prescribed for andropause with reduced sexual desire, premature ejaculation, and erectile dysfunction.

- Selenium metallicum: Used for andropause with weakness, fatigue, and sexual debility.

- Acidum phosphoricum: This remedy is helpful for andropause with mental and physical exhaustion, including cases of sexual weakness.

Oligospermia (Low Sperm Count):

- Agnus castus: Used for oligospermia with reduced sexual desire, premature ejaculation, and erectile dysfunction.

- Lycopodium clavatum: Prescribed for oligospermia accompanied by hormonal imbalances, erectile dysfunction, and premature ejaculation.

- Selenium metallicum: This remedy is helpful for sexual weakness, exhaustion, and oligospermia.

- Acidum phosphoricum: Used for mental and physical exhaustion, including cases of oligospermia.

- Aurum metallicum: Prescribed for depression, anxiety, and oligospermia related to emotional stress.

Insomnia:

- Coffea cruda: Prescribed for insomnia with a busy, active mind and restlessness.

- Nux vomica: Used for insomnia due to overwork, stress, and digestive issues.

- Passiflora incarnata: This remedy is beneficial for insomnia with a restless mind and difficulty falling asleep.

- Chamomilla: Used for insomnia with irritability and sensitivity to pain.

- Ignatia amara: This remedy is helpful for insomnia due to grief, emotional stress, and suppressed emotions.

Pneumonia:

- Bryonia alba: Prescribed for pneumonia with sharp, stitching chest pain aggravated by movement.

- Phosphorus: Used for pneumonia with weakness, hoarseness, and tightness in the chest.

- Antimonium tartaricum: This remedy is beneficial for pneumonia with a rattling cough and difficulty breathing.

- Hepar sulphuris calcareum: Used for pneumonia with extreme sensitivity to cold air and cough with yellow, offensive-smelling mucus.

- Lycopodium clavatum: This remedy is helpful for pneumonia with a bloated abdomen, gas, and respiratory issues.

Testicular Torsion:

- Belladonna: Prescribed for testicular torsion with sudden, intense pain, redness, and heat in the scrotum.

- Colocynthis: Used for testicular torsion with cramping, shooting pain, and relief from bending forward.

- Arnica montana: This remedy is beneficial for testicular torsion with soreness, bruised feeling, and discomfort in the scrotum.

- Hamamelis virginiana: Used for testicular torsion with bruised, sore sensation and bluish discoloration.

- Rhus Toxicodendron: Prescribed for testicular torsion with pain, stiffness, and relief from movement.

Coronary Artery Disease (CAD):

- Crataegus oxyacantha: This remedy is used for CAD to support heart health and improve blood circulation.

- Arnica Montana: Prescribed for CAD with a feeling of heaviness and bruised pain in the chest.

- Cactus grandiflorus: Used for CAD with tightness, constriction, and anxiety about the heart.

- Aurum metallicum: This remedy is beneficial for CAD with depression, anxiety, and a sense of hopelessness.

- Digitalis purpurea: Used for CAD with weak, irregular heartbeat and breathlessness.

Diverticulitis:

- Colocynthis: Prescribed for diverticulitis with severe cramping, colicky abdominal pain, and relief from pressure.

- Nux vomica: Used for diverticulitis with bloating, constipation, and irritability.

- Lycopodium clavatum: This remedy benefits diverticulitis with bloating, gas, and indigestion.

- Phosphorus: Prescribed for diverticulitis with abdominal burning pain and diarrhea.

- Mercurius corrosivus: Used for diverticulitis with intense abdominal pain and tenesmus (straining to pass stools).

Peptic Ulcer Disease:

- Argentum nitricum: This remedy is used for peptic ulcers with burning pain in the stomach and a craving for sweets.

- Nux vomica: Prescribed for peptic ulcers with indigestion, bloating, and irritability.

- Carbo vegetabilis: Used for peptic ulcers with a feeling of fullness and flatulence after eating.

- Phosphorus: This remedy is beneficial for peptic ulcers with a burning sensation and vomiting of undigested food.

- Kali bichromicum: Prescribed for peptic ulcers with a feeling of a lump in the stomach and vomiting of stringy mucus.

Psoriasis:

- Arsenicum album: Used for psoriasis with burning, itching, and dry, scaly skin.

- Sulphur: This remedy benefits psoriasis with intense itching and burning sensations.

- Graphites: Prescribed for psoriasis with thick, cracked, and oozing skin.

- Rhus Toxicodendron: Used for psoriasis with red, swollen, and itchy skin, worsened by cold and damp weather.

- Kali arsenicosis: This remedy is helpful for psoriasis with scaling, flaky skin, and intense itching.

Melasma (Chloasma):

- Thuja occidentalis: Used for melasma with dark, greenish-brown spots on the skin.

- Sulphur: This remedy is beneficial for melasma with dark, red, or brown spots on the skin.

- Natrum muriaticum: Prescribed for melasma with brown patches on the forehead, cheeks, and upper lip.

- Berberis aquifolium: Used for melasma with dark spots and acne-like eruptions on the skin.

Hair Loss (Male Pattern Baldness):

- Acidum fluoricum: This remedy is used for hair loss with excessive falling out of hair.

- Phosphoricum acidum: Prescribed for hair loss due to grief, sadness, or emotional shock.

- Lycopodium clavatum: Used for hair loss with hormonal imbalances and premature graying of hair.

- Thuja occidentalis: This remedy is beneficial for hair loss with brittle hair and dandruff.

- Natrum muriaticum: Prescribed for hair loss related to hormonal imbalances and dandruff.

Gout:

- Colchicum autumnale: Used for gout with intense pain, swelling, and burning in the affected joints.

- Ledum palustre: Prescribed for gout with swollen, pale, and cold joints.

- Benzoicum acidum: This remedy is helpful for gout with strong-smelling urine and intense joint pain.

- Urtica urens: Used for gout with burning, stinging pains, and skin eruptions.

- Sulphur: This remedy benefits gout with burning, itching, and hot feet.

Liver Cirrhosis

- Carduus marianus: Prescribed for liver cirrhosis with abdominal fullness, discomfort, and enlarged liver.

- Chelidonium majus: Used for liver cirrhosis with jaundice, pain in the right upper abdomen, and yellow-coated tongue.

- Lycopodium clavatum: This remedy benefits liver cirrhosis with bloating, gas, and constipation.

- Nux vomica: Prescribed for liver cirrhosis with a tendency to overindulge in rich food, alcohol, and stimulants.

- China officinalis: Used for liver cirrhosis with weakness, pale complexion, and anemia.

Parkinson's Disease:

- Agaricus muscarius: Prescribed for Parkinson's disease with trembling and jerking movements.

- Gelsemium sempervirens: Used for Parkinson's disease with weakness, tremors, and dizziness.

- Zincum metallicum: Used for Parkinson's disease with restlessness, twitching, and limb weakness.

- Lycopodium clavatum: This remedy benefits Parkinson's disease with stiffness, trembling, and digestive issues.

- Causticum: Prescribed for Parkinson's disease with stiffness, difficulty swallowing, and emotional sensitivity.

- Baryta carbonica: Used for Parkinson's disease in elderly individuals with cognitive decline and weakness.

Autism Spectrum Disorder (ASD):

- Stramonium: Prescribed for ASD with violent outbursts, intense fears, and behavioral disturbances.

- Carcinosinum: Used for ASD with sensitivity, anxiety, and emotional vulnerability.

- Tuberculinum aviary: This remedy benefits ASD with restlessness, impulsiveness, and excitability.

- Baryta carbonica: Used for ASD in individuals who are shy, socially anxious, and slow to develop.

- Hyoscyamus niger: This remedy is helpful for ASD with talkativeness, jealousy, and impulsiveness.

Erectile Dysfunction (ED):

- Agnus castus: Prescribed for erectile dysfunction with reduced sexual desire and depression.

- Lycopodium clavatum: Used for ED with hormonal imbalances, premature ejaculation, and performance anxiety.

- Selenium metallicum: This remedy is beneficial for sexual weakness, exhaustion, and ED.

- Acidum phosphoricum: Used for mental and physical exhaustion, including cases of ED.

- Caladium seguinum: This remedy is helpful for ED with sexual desire but a weak erection.

Benign Prostatic Hyperplasia (BPH):

- Sabal serrulata: Prescribed for BPH with difficulty in initiating urination, weak stream, and frequent urination.

- Conium maculatum: Used for BPH with a sensation of fullness and a need to urinate at night.

- Pulsatilla pratensis: This remedy is beneficial for BPH with a frequent urge to urinate, especially at night.

- Thuja occidentalis: Used for BPH with urinary hesitancy, dribbling, and interrupted urine flow.

- Chimaphila umbellata: Prescribed for BPH with painful urination, difficulty in passing urine, and residual urine.

Obsessive-Compulsive Disorder (OCD):

- Arsenicum album: Used for OCD with anxiety, restlessness, and obsessive thoughts about cleanliness or health.

- Natrum muriaticum: This remedy is beneficial for OCD related to suppressed emotions and obsessive thoughts about past events.

- Anacardium orientale: Prescribed for OCD with a feeling of a split personality, inner conflict, and compulsive behaviors.

- Aurum metallicum: Used for OCD with depression, guilt, and obsessive thoughts about failure.

- Veratrum album: This remedy is helpful for OCD with religious or moral obsessions and rituals.

Alopecia Areata:

- Phosphoricum acidum: Prescribed for alopecia areata due to grief, sadness, or emotional shock.

- Fluoricum acidum: Used for alopecia areata with a tendency to premature hair graying and loss.

- Vinca minor: This remedy benefits alopecia areata with circular bald spots and itchy scalp.

- Silicea: Used for alopecia areata with brittle hair, hair loss, and slow regrowth.

- Natrum muriaticum: This remedy is helpful for hair loss due to hormonal imbalances and dandruff.

Laryngitis:

- Arum triphyllum: Prescribed for laryngitis with a raw, burning sensation and hoarseness.

- Spongia tosta: Used for laryngitis with dry, barking cough and hoarseness.

- Causticum: This remedy benefits laryngitis with a weak, hoarse voice and difficulty speaking.

- Kali bichromicum: Prescribed for laryngitis with stringy mucus and a harsh, barking cough.

- Phosphorus: Used for laryngitis with a hoarse voice, itchy sensation, and dry cough.

Gastritis:

- Nux vomica: Prescribed for gastritis with bloating, flatulence, and indigestion after overeating or spicy foods.

- Arsenicum album: Used for gastritis with burning pain in the stomach, nausea, and anxiety.

- Natrum phosphoricum: This remedy benefits gastritis with acidity, heartburn, and sour belching.

- Robinia pseudoacacia: Used for gastritis with excessive acid production and sour regurgitations.

- Carbo vegetabilis: Prescribed for gastritis with a feeling of fullness, belching, and weak digestion.

Sinusitis:

- Kali bichromicum: Used for sinusitis with thick, stringy nasal discharge and frontal headache.

- Pulsatilla pratensis: Prescribed for sinusitis with yellow-green discharge and a diminished sense of smell.

Hepar sulphuris calcareum: This remedy benefits sinusitis with nasal sensitivity, sore throat, and thick yellow discharge.

Silicea: Used for sinusitis with blocked sinuses, facial pain, and dry nose.

Belladonna: Prescribed for sinusitis with sudden onset, intense symptoms, and throbbing head pain.

Liver Cancer:

- Conium maculatum: Used for liver cancer when there is swelling, induration, and hardness of the glands.

- Carcinosinum: Prescribed for cancer-related symptoms and support in cancer cases.

- Thuja occidentalis: This remedy benefits cancer-related symptoms, skin issues, and hormonal imbalances.

- Hydrastis canadensis: Used for cancer symptoms and general immune support.

- Scrophularia nodosa: Prescribed for swollen glands and cancer-related symptoms.

Chronic Bronchitis:

- Antimonium tartaricum: This remedy is used for chronic bronchitis with a rattling cough, difficult expectoration, and weakness.

- Hepar sulphuris calcareum: Prescribed for chronic bronchitis with sensitivity to cold air, a loose rattling cough, and a desire for warmth.

- Spongia tosta: Used for chronic bronchitis with a dry, barking cough and breathing difficulties.

- Bryonia alba: This remedy benefits chronic bronchitis with a dry, painful cough and aggravation from movement.

- Phosphorus: Prescribed for chronic bronchitis with a hard, dry cough and hoarseness.

Epididymal Cyst:

- Pulsatilla pratensis: Used for epididymal cyst with swelling, pain, and a sensation of fullness in the scrotum.

- Clematis recta: This remedy benefits epididymal cysts with painful swelling and drawing pain in the testicles.

- Conium maculatum: Prescribed for epididymal cyst when there is swelling, induration, and hardness of the glands.

- Rhododendron chrysanthum: Used for epididymal cyst with aching, soreness, and drawing pain in the testicles.

- Silicea: This remedy benefits epididymal cysts with hard, painless nodules in the scrotum.

- Apis mellifica: Prescribed for epididymal cyst with swelling, redness, and stinging pain in the scrotum.

- Clematis vitalba: Used for epididymal cyst with aching, bruised pain in the testicles.

Benign Prostatic Enlargement (BPE) (Benign Prostatic Hyperplasia - BPH):

- Sabal serrulata: This remedy is used for BPE/BPH with difficulty initiating urination, weak stream, and frequent urination.

- Conium maculatum: Prescribed for BPE/BPH with a sensation of fullness and a need to urinate at night.

- Pulsatilla pratensis: Used for BPE/BPH with a frequent urge to urinate, especially at night.

- Thuja occidentalis: This remedy benefits BPE/BPH with urinary hesitancy, dribbling, and interrupted urine flow.

- Chimaphila umbellata: Prescribed for BPE/BPH with painful urination, difficulty in passing urine, and residual urine.

Hypogonadism (Low Testosterone):

- Agnus castus: Used for hypogonadism with reduced sexual desire, weakness, and erectile dysfunction.

- Lycopodium clavatum: This remedy is beneficial for hypogonadism with hormonal imbalances, premature ejaculation, and performance anxiety.

- Selenium metallicum: Prescribed for sexual weakness, exhaustion, and hypogonadism.

- Acidum phosphoricum: Used for mental and physical exhaustion, including cases of hypogonadism.

- Aurum metallicum: This remedy is helpful for depression, anxiety, and hypogonadism related to emotional stress.

Testicular Cancer:

- Conium maculatum: Prescribed for testicular cancer when there is swelling, induration, and hardness of the glands.

- Carcinosinum: Used for cancer-related symptoms and support in cancer cases.

- Thuja occidentalis: This remedy benefits cancer-related symptoms, skin issues, and hormonal imbalances.

- Hydrastis canadensis: Used for cancer symptoms and general immune support.

- Scrophularia nodosa: Prescribed for swollen glands and cancer-related symptoms.

Polycystic Ovary Syndrome (PCOS) in Men (Stein-Leventhal Syndrome):

- Pulsatilla pratensis: This remedy is used for PCOS in men with hormonal imbalances, emotional sensitivity, and changeable nature of symptoms.

- Sepia officinalis: Prescribed for PCOS in men with suppressed emotions, fatigue, and irritability.

- Lachesis mutus: Used for PCOS in men with left-sided symptoms, heat intolerance, and mood swings.

- Phosphorus: This remedy is beneficial for PCOS in men with a desire for cold drinks, sensitive to light, and easily fatigued.

- Natrum muriaticum: Prescribed for PCOS in men with emotional suppression, sadness, and salt cravings.

Prostatitis (Chronic Nonbacterial):

- Pulsatilla pratensis: Used for chronic nonbacterial prostatitis with a sensation of fullness, heaviness, and discomfort in the pelvis.

- Thuja occidentalis: This remedy benefits chronic nonbacterial prostatitis with urinary hesitancy, dribbling, and painful urination.

- Sarsaparilla officinalis: Prescribed for chronic nonbacterial prostatitis with burning pain at the end of urination and kidney colic.

- Staphysagria: Used for chronic nonbacterial prostatitis with a history of suppressed emotions and sensitivity.

- Clematis recta: This remedy is helpful for chronic nonbacterial prostatitis with a frequent urge to urinate and difficulty passing urine.

Erectile Dysfunction (ED) due to Psychological Factors:

- Agnus castus: Prescribed for ED with reduced sexual desire and depression.

- Lycopodium clavatum: Used for ED with hormonal imbalances, premature ejaculation, and performance anxiety.

- Selenium metallicum: This remedy is beneficial for sexual weakness, exhaustion, and ED.

- Acidum phosphoricum: Used for mental and physical exhaustion, including cases of ED.

- Caladium seguinum: This remedy is helpful for ED with sexual desire but a weak erection.

Chapter 4: The Vital Role of First Aid and the Complementary Potential of Homeopathy in Non-Critical Situations

First aid is a cornerstone of emergency response, providing initial care to injured or unwell individuals before professional medical assistance becomes available. The fundamental objectives of first aid encompass preserving life, preventing deterioration of the condition, and expediting the process of recovery. Proficiency in administering first aid is desirable and imperative, as it empowers individuals to respond promptly and effectively during moments of crisis, ultimately playing a pivotal role in determining outcomes for those in need.

Benefits of First Aid:

Immediate Response

One of the most significant benefits of first aid is its capacity to offer immediate assistance at the scene of an incident. It bridges the critical gap between the occurrence of an injury or ailment and the arrival of medical professionals. This rapid response can significantly impact the individual's chances of survival and recovery.

Injury Mitigation

Properly administered first aid techniques have the potential to prevent minor injuries from escalating into more severe conditions. Swift action, such as immobilizing a fractured bone, can prevent further harm and reduce the long-term impact of the damage.

Preservation of Life

In dire situations, the quick and appropriate application of first aid can make the difference between life and death. Essential interventions like cardiopulmonary resuscitation (CPR) or stopping severe bleeding can be lifesaving until advanced medical help arrives.

Acceleration of Recovery

Immediate care through first aid not only prevents the condition from worsening but can also expedite the recovery process. For instance, cooling a burn promptly can limit tissue damage and aid faster healing.

Confidence Building

Acquiring knowledge of first aid boosts confidence in individuals, enabling them to take charge during emergencies. This empowerment translates to more effective assistance and better decision-making in high-pressure situations.

Complication Minimization

Timely first aid can prevent complications that might arise due to delays in receiving medical attention. Treating a wound promptly, for example, reduces the risk of infection and ensures proper healing.

Support for Medical Personnel

In specific scenarios, administering first aid can stabilize the patient's condition until professional medical help becomes available. This support is precious when immediate access to medical facilities is limited.

Importance of First Aid Knowledge:

Preparedness for Emergency

Proficiency in first aid equips individuals with the skills needed to respond effectively to a wide range of emergencies. Whether it's a car accident, a sudden cardiac arrest, or an accidental fall, those trained in first aid can provide critical assistance until medical professionals arrive.

Amplified Safety

Knowledge of first aid fosters a safer environment, not only for the person administering aid but also for those around them. Prompt intervention can prevent accidents from escalating and causing harm to multiple individuals.

Contributing to Community Health

Individuals well-versed in first aid play an active role in enhancing the overall health and safety of their communities. Their ability to respond promptly during emergencies can minimize the impact of injuries and ailments on a broader scale.

Time-Sensitive Response

There are situations where time is of the essence, such as during a heart attack or a choking incident. Immediate first aid intervention can stabilize the individual's condition and prevent further harm until professional medical assistance is available.

Remote Area Assistance

In remote locations or during natural disasters, access to medical help may be delayed. First aid skills become indispensable in such contexts, as they ensure that immediate care is available even in challenging circumstances.

Support for Non-Critical Injuries

First aid knowledge extends beyond life-threatening situations. Minor injuries like cuts, bruises, sprains, and burns are common occurrences that can be effectively managed with the application of first aid techniques.

Complementary Homeopathy in Non-Critical First Aid Situations:

Homeopathy, a holistic medical approach, operates on the principle of "like cures like." It involves using highly diluted substances derived from natural sources to stimulate the body's inherent healing mechanisms. While homeopathy should not replace conventional first aid practices, it can offer a complementary approach to managing certain non-critical conditions.

Several notable examples include:

Arnica montana

This homeopathic remedy is frequently employed to address bruising, sprains, and muscle soreness. It is believed to aid in reducing swelling and promoting the healing process following minor injuries.

Calendula officinalis

Often used for cuts, scrapes, and superficial wounds, this homeopathic remedy may contribute to wound healing and lower the risk of infection.

-Api

smellifica

In the case of insect bites and stings, this remedy is thought to alleviate pain, swelling, and redness, providing relief to the affected individual.

Hypericum perforatum:

Utilized for nerve injuries, such as pinched fingers or toes, this homeopathic remedy is believed to alleviate shooting pains and discomfort associated with nerve-related injuries.

It's important to emphasize that homeopathy should be regarded as a supplementary tool within the realm of first aid. It is not a substitute for prompt medical attention, particularly in situations where life is at risk or when injuries are severe. In such cases, seeking professional medical help remains paramount.

By combining the principles of first aid with the potential benefits of homeopathy in non-critical situations, individuals can enhance their capacity to provide effective and comprehensive care during times of need.

Disclaimer

Please read the following terms and conditions carefully before proceeding.

General Information Purposes Only: The information provided in the following is for general informational and entertainment purposes only. All information is provided in good faith; however, the author makes no representation or warranty of any kind, express or implied, regarding the accuracy, adequacy, validity, reliability, availability, or completeness of any information on the following.

Not Medical Advice: The content provided below is not intended to be a substitute for professional medical advice, diagnosis, or treatment. Always seek the advice of your physician or other qualified health providers with any questions you may have regarding a medical condition or health concerns.

No Doctor-Patient Relationship: reading the below

information does not constitute the establishment of a doctor-patient relationship. Any health information communicated is not an endorsement, diagnosis, or treatment regimen.

Professional Assistance: You must not rely on the information below as an alternative to medical advice from your doctor or other professional healthcare providers. If you believe you are experiencing any medical condition, you should seek immediate medical attention from a licensed healthcare provider.

Risks of Self-Diagnosis: Self-diagnosis can lead to harm, and it is critical that healthcare professionals perform diagnosis and treatment.

Limitation of Warranties: The medical information provided is "as is" without any representations or warranties, express or implied. The author no representations or warranties concerning the medical information.

Liability: You agree to release the offer from any and all liability and to hold him harmless from any legal claims related to the medical information provided.

Contact a Doctor: Do not disregard, avoid, or delay obtaining medical advice from a qualified healthcare provider because of something you may have read in this book or below.

You do understand and agree to the terms of this disclaimer. If you do not agree with these terms, you are not

authorized to obtain information from or otherwise proceed.

Cuts and Scrapes:

• First Aid: For minor cuts and scrapes, it is crucial to clean the wound gently with mild soap and water to prevent infection. After cleaning, applying an over-the-counter antibiotic ointment can further protect against bacteria. Covering the wound with a sterile bandage safeguards it from external contaminants and friction that could delay healing.

•Homeopathic:

• Calendula ointment: Derived from the marigold plant, known for accelerating wound healing and reducing inflammation. It possesses antiseptic properties and helps minimize scar formation.

• Hypericum perforatum: Known as St. John's Wort, effective for cuts with nerve damage. It has nerve-healing properties and is used for injuries in nerve-rich areas.

Bruises:

• First Aid: When dealing with bruises, applying a cold compress or ice pack to the bruised area within the first 24 hours can help minimize swelling and pain. This constricts blood vessels and reduces blood flow to the area, which helps in reducing the bruise's size and severity. Resting the affected area can also prevent further trauma to the injured blood vessels.

• Homeopathic:

• Arnica montana: A primary remedy for bruises, reducing swelling and decreasing discoloration. It facilitates blood circulation and helps in reabsorption of blood from bruised tissues.

• Bellis perennis: Used for deeper tissue injuries and bruises, especially with soreness. Helpful in cases where Arnica does not suffice.

Sprains and Strains:

• First Aid: The R.I.C.E. method (Rest, Ice, Compression, Elevation) is the standard approach for managing sprains and strains. Resting allows for healing, applying ice reduces inflammation, compression supports the injured area, and elevation reduces swelling by encouraging fluid drainage.

• Homeopathic:

• Ruta graveolens: Useful for injuries to ligaments, tendons, and bone linings. Relieves pain and aids in healing strain or sprain injuries.

• Symphytum officinale: Known as 'knitbone', aids in the healing of sprained ligaments and tendons, and accelerates bone healing.

Sunburn:

• First Aid: For sunburn, cooling the affected skin with a cool bath or compress provides relief. Applying aloe vera gel soothes the burn, and staying hydrated is vital for recovery and maintaining skin hydration.

• Homeopathic:

• Cantharis: Used for first-degree burns and sunburns, reducing burning sensation and promoting healing. Effective for burns better with cold applications.

• Sulphur: Suitable for sunburns that are itchy and worsen with heat. Also used for various skin conditions.

Insect Bites and Stings:

• First Aid: In the case of insect bites and stings, it's important to remove the stinger if present, clean the area, and apply a cold pack to reduce swelling and itching. Refraining from scratching the bite area is crucial to prevent further irritation and potential infection.

• Homeopathic:

• Apis mellifica: Effective for bites causing redness, swelling, and itching, particularly when there is edema and stinging pain.

• Ledum palustre: Indicated for puncture wounds and animal and insect bites. Effective when the affected area is cold and relieved by cold applications.

Minor Burns:

• First Aid: Immediate cooling of the burn with cold water can minimize tissue damage and pain. After cooling, applying an antibiotic ointment and covering with a sterile bandage creates a protective barrier, preventing infection and promoting a moist healing environment.

• Homeopathic:

• Urtica urens: Used for first-degree burns with redness and intense burning. Reduces burning sensation and supports tissue regeneration.

• Causticum: Suitable for burns causing blistering, helping to relieve pain associated with burn injuries.

Allergic Reactions (mild):

• First Aid: For mild allergic reactions, the first step is to remove the allergen if possible. Taking an over-the-counter antihistamine may help alleviate the symptoms. It's also important to avoid further exposure to the allergen to prevent additional reactions.

• Homeopathic:

• Histaminum: Derived from histamine, used for allergic reactions, helping to regulate the body's histamine response.

• Urtica urens: Effective for allergic reactions resembling nettle rash, especially with intense itching.

Nausea and Vomiting:

• First Aid: Managing nausea and vomiting involves sipping small amounts of water, avoiding solid foods initially, and resting. Incorporating ginger, peppermint tea, or dry crackers can also provide relief.

• Homeopathic:

• Nux vomica: Made from the strychnine tree seeds, often used for nausea and vomiting associated with overeating or stress.

• Ipecacuanha: Effective for persistent nausea and vomiting, especially when accompanied by excessive salivation. Ipecacuanha is also used for coughs with nausea.

Muscle Cramps:

• First Aid: Gently stretching and massaging the affected muscle can provide immediate relief for muscle cramps. Applying a warm compress can help relax the muscle and ease the pain. Maintaining proper hydration and electrolyte balance is also crucial in preventing muscle cramps.

• Homeopathic:

• Magnesia phosphorica: A remedy for muscle cramps and spasms, particularly in the legs. Known for its ability to relieve cramps and pain.

• Cuprum metallicum: Useful for severe muscle cramps and spasms, especially in the lower limbs and relieved by warmth.

Minor Eye Irritations:

• First Aid: Flushing the irritated eye with clean water is a primary step in providing relief. This helps remove any foreign particles or irritants. If irritation persists or if the eye has been exposed to a chemical, seeking medical help is essential.

• Homeopathic:

• Euphrasia: Commonly known as eyebright, used for eye irritation associated with colds or allergies. It helps relieve redness, irritation, and watery discharge.

• Belladonna: Indicated for red, swollen eyes with a sensation of heat, often used for acute conditions and sudden eye irritations.

Nosebleeds:

• First Aid: For nosebleeds, sitting upright and leaning forward slightly while pinching the soft part of the nose for several minutes can help stop the bleeding. It's important to avoid vigorous nose-blowing or inserting anything into the nose, as this can exacerbate the bleeding.

• Homeopathic:

• Ferrum phosphoricum: Used for nosebleeds resulting from minor injuries. Believed to support blood clotting and strengthen blood vessels.

• Hamamelis: Known as Witch Hazel, effective for nosebleeds with a sensation of fullness or bursting. Often used for venous bleeding and varicose veins.

Splinters:

• First Aid: Using clean tweezers to gently remove the splinter is the first step. The area should then be cleaned, and an antibiotic ointment and bandage should be applied to help prevent infection. Proper removal and care are important to prevent complications.

• Homeopathic:

• Silicea: Assists in the expulsion of foreign objects like splinters, indicated when splinters are lodged deep in the skin and are painful.

• Hepar sulphuris calcareum: Useful for deep, painful splinters, and for infections. Helps the body expel the splinter and can be used when there is pus or infection.

Mild Burns from Hot Objects (e.g., touching a hot pan):

• First Aid: Promptly cooling the affected area under cold running water minimizes tissue damage and alleviates pain. It is essential to cool the burn for several minutes to reduce the heat in the tissue and alleviate pain. Avoid applying ice directly to the burn as it can cause further damage to the skin.

• Homeopathic: Cantharis, derived from the Spanish fly, is believed to help with pain and blistering resulting from minor burns caused by hot objects. It's thought to assist in reducing the intensity of burn-related discomfort. Additional Homeopathic Remedy: Phosphorus can be beneficial for burns that feel better with cold applications and have a burning sensation.

Indigestion:

• First Aid: Alleviating indigestion involves avoiding heavy, spicy, and greasy foods. Drinking ginger or peppermint tea can help soothe the stomach and improve digestion by promoting the flow of digestive juices. Eating smaller, more frequent meals and avoiding lying down after eating can also provide relief.

• Homeopathic: Carbo vegetabilis, sourced from vegetable charcoal, is suggested for bloating and flatulence associated with indigestion. It's believed to help ease gas buildup and enhance digestion. Additional Homeopathic Remedy: Lycopodium is indicated for indigestion with bloating, especially in the lower abdomen and often associated with gas.

Mild Heat Exhaustion:

• First Aid: Combating mild heat exhaustion includes moving to a cooler area, drinking cool water, and resting. Applying a damp cloth to the forehead and neck can help regulate body temperature. It's important to rest in a cool environment and slowly rehydrate.

• Homeopathic: Gelsemium, prepared from the yellow jasmine plant, is believed to provide relief from weakness and fatigue linked to heat exhaustion. It's thought to support the body in recovering from physical and emotional stress. Additional Homeopathic Remedy: Belladonna can be useful in heat exhaustion, especially if there is a rapid onset and the person feels hot and flushed.

Minor Gastrointestinal Upset (e.g., traveler's diarrhea):

• First Aid: Addressing traveler's diarrhea involves staying hydrated with oral rehydration solutions and avoiding spicy and greasy foods. It is crucial to replace lost fluids and electrolytes to prevent dehydration. Resting and avoiding dehydration are crucial.

• Homeopathic: Arsenicum album, derived from arsenic trioxide, is considered for cases of diarrhea accompanied by weakness and restlessness. It's believed to aid in addressing gastrointestinal upset and discomfort. Additional Homeopathic Remedy: Podophyllum is often used for diarrhea that is profuse and gushing.

Minor Emotional Shock or Trauma:

• First Aid: Providing comfort and support to individuals experiencing emotional shock or trauma is crucial. Encouraging deep breathing, providing a safe space for expression, and seeking professional help if needed are essential steps. It is important to listen without judgment and offer a calming presence.

• Homeopathic: Ignatia amara, sourced from the St. Ignatius bean, is used to address emotional distress, grief, or shock. It's believed to support emotional balance and resilience during challenging times. Additional Homeopathic Remedy: Aconitum napellus is beneficial for acute shock and fear, especially following a traumatic event.

Minor Dehydration:

• First Aid: Minor dehydration can occur due to inadequate fluid intake, excessive sweating, or illness. Drink plenty of fluids, especially water or oral rehydration solutions, to restore fluid balance and prevent dehydration. Rehydrating with electrolyte-rich solutions can be beneficial, especially after physical activity or illness.

• Homeopathic: Veratrum album, prepared from white hellebore, is suggested for cases of profuse, watery diarrhea leading to dehydration. This remedy is believed to help regulate fluid loss and maintain electrolyte balance. Additional Homeopathic Remedy: China officinalis can be helpful for dehydration, particularly when it is due to excessive fluid loss, like in diarrhea or sweating.

Motion Sickness:

• First Aid: Motion sickness can cause nausea, vomiting, and dizziness during travel. To alleviate symptoms, focus on the horizon, avoid reading or using screens, and consider acupressure wristbands or ginger supplements to ease nausea. Taking slow, deep breaths and ensuring proper ventilation in the vehicle can also help reduce discomfort.

• Homeopathic: Cocculus indicus, prepared from Indian cockle, is recommended for addressing dizziness, nausea, and vomiting caused by motion sickness. It's believed to stabilize the inner ear and alleviate associated symptoms, making it a potential natural option for relief. Additional Homeopathic Remedy: Tabacum is often used for severe motion sickness, especially when there is cold sweat and a feeling of extreme nausea.

Mild Food Poisoning:

• First Aid: Mild food poisoning can result from consuming contaminated food or water. Resting and staying hydrated with clear fluids like water, clear broths, and oral rehydration solutions is essential. Avoid solid foods for a few hours to allow the stomach to settle, then gradually reintroduce bland, easily digestible foods as symptoms improve.

• Homeopathic: Arsenicum album, derived from arsenic trioxide, can assist with diarrhea, vomiting, and weakness due to food poisoning. It's believed to help restore digestive balance and alleviate associated discomfort. Additional Homeopathic Remedy: Podophyllum can be beneficial for food poisoning, especially with profuse diarrhea and cramping.

Allergic Skin Reactions (e.g., hives):

• First Aid: Minor allergic skin reactions such as hives can be triggered by allergens like certain foods, medications, or insect bites. Applying a cool compress to the affected area can help alleviate itching and reduce inflammation. Avoid scratching, as it can worsen symptoms. Over-the-counter antihistamines may be taken as directed to provide relief.

• Homeopathic: Urtica urens, prepared from the common nettle, is commonly used for hives and skin itching. It's believed to have anti-inflammatory properties and aid in addressing allergic reactions. Additional Homeopathic Remedy: Apis mellifica is effective for hives, especially when there is swelling, stinging pain, and itching that improves with cold applications.

Foreign Object in the Eye:

• First Aid: A minor foreign object in the eye, such as dust or an eyelash, can cause irritation and discomfort. Rinse the eye with clean water or saline solution to flush out the foreign object. Blinking several times may help dislodge the object from the eye. If irritation persists, seeking medical attention is advised.

• Homeopathic: Euphrasia, commonly known as eyebright, is used to address eye irritation caused by foreign objects. It's believed to provide relief and promote eye comfort. Additional Homeopathic Remedy: Aconitum napellus can be used when there is sudden intense pain or discomfort in the eye, often from exposure to wind or cold air.

Acid Indigestion:

• First Aid: Mild acid indigestion can result from consuming acidic foods or excessive caffeine. To alleviate discomfort, avoid acidic foods and beverages, drink water or milk to neutralize excess stomach acid, and consider using antacids if needed. Eating smaller, more frequent meals and avoiding lying down after eating can also help.

• Homeopathic: Nux vomica, derived from the strychnine tree, is recommended for acid indigestion accompanied by symptoms like bloating and flatulence. It's believed to help restore digestive harmony and address discomfort caused by dietary indiscretions. Additional Homeopathic Remedy: Robinia is often used for acid indigestion with sour belching and burning in the stomach.

Sunstroke:

• First Aid: Mild sunstroke, resulting from prolonged exposure to heat, can cause headaches, dizziness, and dehydration. Move the person to a cool, shaded area to lower body temperature, apply cool compresses to the forehead and neck to dissipate heat, and give them small sips of water to stay hydrated. Resting in a comfortable position is important.

• Homeopathic: Glonoinum, prepared from nitroglycerin, is suggested for throbbing headaches and heat-related symptoms associated with mild sunstroke. It's believed to support vascular dilation and improve blood circulation, aiding in relief from heat-related discomfort. Additional Homeopathic Remedy: Belladonna can be beneficial in cases of sunstroke where there is a sudden onset of symptoms, redness of the face, and a feeling of throbbing in the head.

Minor Foot Fungus (Athlete's Foot):

• First Aid: Athlete's foot is a fungal infection that commonly affects the feet. Keeping the feet clean and dry, using antifungal creams or sprays as directed to control the infection, and avoiding wearing tight shoes that may exacerbate moisture buildup are important. Changing socks frequently and letting your feet breathe can aid in recovery.

• Homeopathic: Sulphur, prepared from the element sulphur, can assist with itchy and burning foot fungus. It's believed to address fungal infections and related discomfort. Additional Homeopathic Remedy: Graphites is often recommended for foot fungus, especially when there are cracks and soreness in the skin.

Mild Nose Allergies (Allergic Rhinitis):

• First Aid: Mild allergic rhinitis, commonly known as hay fever, can cause symptoms like a runny or stuffy nose, sneezing, and watery eyes. To manage symptoms, avoid allergens, use saline nasal sprays to keep nasal passages moist, and consider over-the-counter antihistamines if needed. Creating an allergen-free indoor environment and using air purifiers can also help reduce exposure to allergens.

• Homeopathic: Allium cepa, prepared from red onion, is recommended for addressing symptoms of runny nose and watery eyes associated with allergic rhinitis. It's believed to have anti-allergic properties and may provide relief from common allergic reactions. Additional Homeopathic Remedy: Natrum muriaticum can be effective for allergic rhinitis, especially when symptoms include sneezing, watery discharge, and a sensation of dryness.

First Aid: Using a humidifier in dry environments helps maintain skin moisture. Aloe vera gel can provide soothing relief.

Homeopathic: Graphites, derived from graphite minerals, might be chosen for persistent dry skin.

Corns or Calluses:

• First Aid: Corns and calluses are thickened areas of skin that develop due to friction or pressure, often on the feet. To manage mild cases, regularly soaking the affected area in warm water helps soften the skin, making it easier to gently exfoliate the buildup using a pumice stone. Afterward, applying a moisturizing cream can keep the skin supple and prevent further hardening. Wearing comfortable, well-fitting shoes and using protective pads can prevent recurrence by reducing pressure on the sensitive areas.

• Homeopathic: Antimonium crudum, derived from antimony trisulfide, is suggested for addressing painful corns and calluses. It's believed to assist in addressing skin conditions and promoting healing.

• Additional Homeopathic Remedy: Thuja occidentalis is often used for corns and calluses that have a rough, cauliflower-like appearance and can be sensitive to touch.

Tinnitus (Ringing in the Ears):

• First Aid: Tinnitus is often perceived as ringing, buzzing, or other noises in the ears when no external sound is present. To manage mild tinnitus, reducing exposure to loud noises is crucial to prevent aggravation. Stress-reducing techniques such as meditation, deep breathing exercises, and ensuring adequate, quality sleep can also be helpful in managing symptoms. Regular exercise and a healthy diet can contribute to overall well-being and may reduce the severity of tinnitus symptoms.

• Homeopathic: Salicylicum acidum, prepared from salicylic acid, is recommended for tinnitus accompanied by noises resembling roaring, ringing, or hissing. It's believed to provide relief from auditory disturbances.

• Additional Homeopathic Remedy: Chininum sulphuricum is often used for tinnitus with a sensation of ringing or roaring, sometimes associated with hearing loss or vertigo.

Mild Diaper Rash:

• First Aid: Frequent diaper changes are essential to prevent moisture buildup, which is a common cause of diaper rash. Opt for diapers that offer good airflow and absorb moisture effectively. After gently cleaning the area during each diaper change, applying a barrier cream containing zinc oxide can help create a protective layer against moisture. Allowing the baby's skin to air dry before putting on a new diaper can accelerate healing. Using fragrance-free wipes or just water for cleaning can also help avoid further irritation.

• Homeopathic: Chamomilla's anti-inflammatory properties can help alleviate diaper rash discomfort.

• Additional Homeopathic Remedy: Calendula, known for its healing and soothing properties, can be effective in treating mild diaper rash, promoting skin repair and reducing inflammation.

Allergic Reactions to Medications:

• First Aid: If a mild allergic reaction to a medication occurs, such as itching or a mild rash, the first step is to stop the medication and consult a healthcare professional. It's important to monitor the symptoms closely, as allergic reactions can sometimes worsen. Over-the-counter antihistamines can be used to relieve symptoms like itching and hives. For anaphylactic reactions, which are severe and can include difficulty breathing, immediate medical attention is required.

• Homeopathic: Apis mellifica, derived from honeybees, has been used in homeopathy for skin conditions with swelling, itching, and stinging sensations.

• Additional Homeopathic Remedy: Urtica urens is another remedy that can be effective for allergic reactions, particularly for hives and itching that resemble nettle rash.

Mild Food Allergies (e.g., hives or itching):

• First Aid: Identifying and avoiding trigger foods is crucial for managing mild food allergies. Symptoms such as hives, itching, or mild swelling can often be managed with over-the-counter antihistamines. Keeping an allergy journal can help identify potential triggers. It's important to read food labels carefully to avoid allergenic ingredients. In cases where symptoms involve difficulty breathing or swelling of the throat, immediate medical attention is necessary, as these could indicate a more severe allergic reaction.

• Homeopathic: Urtica urens, prepared from the common nettle plant, has been used for its potential to relieve itching and hives associated with mild food allergies.

• Additional Homeopathic Remedy: Natrum muriaticum can be effective for allergies, especially when there is sneezing and watery discharge from the eyes and nose, resembling symptoms of hay fever.

Chapped Lips:

• First Aid: Chapped lips can be caused by various factors, including cold weather, wind, dehydration, and sun exposure. To prevent and treat chapped lips, it is essential to stay hydrated by drinking plenty of water. Using a lip balm with SPF protection can help protect the lips from sun damage. Applying a natural moisturizer like honey or coconut oil can also soothe and heal dry, cracked lips. Avoid licking your lips, as saliva can exacerbate dryness. In cold or windy weather, covering your lips with a scarf can provide additional protection.

• Homeopathic: Petroleum, derived from refined mineral oil, is a common homeopathic remedy for dry, cracked skin and lips.

- Additional Homeopathic Remedy: Calendula, known for its healing properties, can also be used to soothe and repair chapped lips, especially when there is inflammation and soreness.

Sore Muscles from Exercise:

- First Aid: After strenuous exercise, applying a warm compress or taking a warm bath can help increase blood flow to sore muscles, aiding in recovery and reducing stiffness. Gentle stretching and light activity can maintain muscle flexibility and prevent further soreness. Hydration and proper nutrition, including adequate protein intake, are essential for muscle recovery.

- Homeopathic: Bryonia, made from the white bryony plant, is suggested for soreness that's worsened by movement.

- Arnica, derived from the arnica plant, is renowned for reducing muscle pain and inflammation post-exertion.

- Additional Homeopathic Remedy: Rhus toxicodendron is often used for muscle soreness that improves with movement, especially when stiffness is prominent upon waking or after prolonged inactivity.

Eye Fatigue from Screen Use:

- First Aid: Eye fatigue from prolonged screen use can be alleviated by following the 20-20-20 rule: every 20 minutes, take a 20-second break to look at something 20 feet away. Adjusting the screen to eye level, reducing glare, and ensuring proper lighting can also reduce eye strain. Using artificial tears or lubricating eye drops can alleviate dryness. Ensuring regular eye examinations can help detect any underlying vision problems that may contribute to eye fatigue.

- Homeopathic: Ruta graveolens, made from the common rue plant, is believed to support eye health and relieve eyestrain associated with reading or screen time.

- Additional Homeopathic Remedy: Cineraria maritima has been traditionally used to relieve eye strain and fatigue, particularly when there is a sensation of dryness or discomfort in the eyes.

Motion-Related Vertigo:

- First Aid: If experiencing vertigo, especially related to motion, it's important to sit or lie down immediately to prevent falls and injuries. Keeping the head still and focusing on a stationary object can help reduce the sensation of spinning. Ginger supplements, acupressure wristbands, or ginger tea might help alleviate symptoms. Avoiding sudden movements and gradually changing positions can also help reduce episodes of vertigo.

- Homeopathic: Cocculus indicus, derived from the Indian cockle, is indicated for dizziness caused by motion sickness or travel.

- Additional Homeopathic Remedy: Conium maculatum is often used in cases of vertigo, especially when the dizziness worsens with turning the head or changing positions.

Peptic Ulcers:

- First Aid: Lifestyle modifications are important in managing mild peptic ulcers. This includes avoiding foods and beverages that can irritate the stomach lining, such as caffeine, spicy foods, and alcohol. Eating smaller, more frequent meals can help minimize discomfort. Over-the-counter antacids can provide temporary relief from ulcer pain. Avoiding smoking and reducing stress can also contribute to healing.

- Homeopathic: Arsenicum album, made from arsenic trioxide, might be used for peptic ulcer symptoms characterized by burning pain and anxiety.

- Additional Homeopathic Remedy: Nux vomica is often considered for ulcers, especially when there is a sensation of discomfort or pressure in the stomach, often worsened by eating.

Restlessness or Hyperactivity:

- First Aid: For individuals experiencing mild restlessness or hyperactivity, incorporating a structured routine with calming activities, such as reading or gentle exercise, can be beneficial. Ensuring adequate sleep, promoting a consistent sleep schedule, and engaging in regular physical activity are important. Reducing exposure to stimulating activities, especially before bedtime, can also help manage hyperactivity and restlessness.

- Homeopathic: Tarentula hispanica, derived from a type of wolf spider, is thought to address restlessness and hyperactivity.

- Additional Homeopathic Remedy: Coffea cruda, prepared from unroasted coffee beans, is often used in homeopathy for individuals with an overactive mind and restlessness, particularly when there is difficulty sleeping due to mental hyperactivity.

Throat Irritation from Coughing:

- First Aid: To soothe minor throat irritation caused by coughing, drinking warm liquids, such as tea with honey, can provide relief. Gargling with warm salt water can help reduce inflammation and discomfort. Using a humidifier in the room, especially during dry seasons, can help keep the throat moist and reduce irritation. Avoiding irritants like smoke and strong fragrances can also prevent further throat irritation.

- Homeopathic: Belladonna, made from the deadly nightshade plant, is suggested for sudden onset of intense throat irritation.

- Additional Homeopathic Remedy: Phosphorus is often recommended for throat irritation that is accompanied by a hoarse, dry cough and a feeling of tightness in
the throat.

Constipation:

- First Aid: Dietary fiber from fruits, vegetables, and whole grains aids digestion and can help relieve mild constipation. Incorporating natural laxatives like prunes, flaxseeds, and psyllium husk into the diet can also be effective. Staying hydrated by drinking plenty of water and engaging in regular physical activity can help stimulate bowel movements. Avoiding excessive use of laxatives is important, as it can lead to dependency.

- Homeopathic: Nux vomica, prepared from the strychnine tree's seeds, is a common choice for constipation, especially when accompanied by frequent, ineffective urges.

- Additional Homeopathic Remedy: Alumina is often used in cases of constipation where there is a lack of urge, and the stool is hard and dry.

Acid Reflux (Heartburn):

- First Aid: Elevating the head of the bed can help prevent stomach acid from flowing back into the esophagus during sleep. Avoiding foods and beverages that trigger acid reflux, such as caffeine, spicy foods, and alcohol, is important. Eating smaller, more frequent meals and not lying down immediately after eating can also help reduce symptoms. Over-the-counter antacids can provide temporary relief.

- Homeopathic: Pulsatilla, made from windflower, is used for heartburn worsened by consuming rich, fatty foods.

- Additional Homeopathic Remedy: Robinia, often used for acid reflux symptoms, is effective especially when there is an acidic or sour taste in the mouth.

Sudden Tooth Sensitivity:

- First Aid: Using toothpaste designed for sensitive teeth can help reduce discomfort. Avoiding extremely hot or cold foods and beverages can help prevent aggravating the sensitivity. Gentle brushing with a soft-bristled toothbrush and avoiding acidic foods can also protect sensitive teeth.

- Homeopathic: Coffea cruda, derived from unroasted coffee beans, is suggested for sudden, sharp tooth pain often triggered by hot or cold stimuli.

- Additional Homeopathic Remedy: Hypericum perforatum is effective for nerve pain, particularly useful when tooth sensitivity is severe and radiates along the nerve path.

Sleep Disturbances (Insomnia):

- First Aid: Establishing a relaxing bedtime routine and creating a comfortable sleep environment can aid in combating insomnia. Techniques such as meditation, deep breathing, or progressive muscle relaxation can promote relaxation and make it easier to fall asleep. Limiting screen time before bed, reducing caffeine intake, and ensuring regular exercise can also improve sleep quality.

- Homeopathic: Coffea cruda is recommended for individuals with an overactive mind interfering with their ability to fall asleep.

- Additional Homeopathic Remedy: Passiflora incarnata is often used in cases of insomnia, particularly when there is restlessness and difficulty in switching off the mind.

Joint Sprain:

First Aid: Applying a compression bandage can reduce swelling. Gentle range-of-motion exercises aid in preventing stiffness during recovery.

Homeopathic: Ruta graveolens, prepared from the rue plant, is indicated for injuries involving ligaments and tendons.

Diaper Rash:

First Aid: Frequent diaper changes are essential to prevent moisture buildup. Opt for diapers with good airflow. Apply a barrier cream containing zinc oxide to create a protective layer. Allowing the baby's skin to air dry can accelerate healing.

Homeopathic: Chamomilla's anti-inflammatory properties can help alleviate diaper rash discomfort. It's important to ensure the baby's diaper area is kept clean and dry to support the healing process.

Food Allergies (e.g., hives or itching):

First Aid: Identifying and avoiding trigger foods is crucial. Mild reactions can be managed with antihistamines, but if symptoms worsen or involve difficulty breathing, seek medical help immediately.

Homeopathic: Urtica urens, prepared from the common nettle plant, has been used for its potential to relieve itching and hives.

Chapped Lips:

First Aid: In addition to moisturizing, drinking water helps maintain skin hydration. Use a lip balm with SPF protection. Applying honey can also help soothe and heal dry lips.

Homeopathic: Petroleum, derived from refined mineral oil, is a common homeopathic remedy for dry, cracked skin and lips.

Sore Muscles from Exercise:

First Aid: Applying a warm compress helps increase blood flow to the sore muscles, aiding recovery. Stretching gently after exercise can prevent stiffness.

Homeopathic: Bryonia, made from the white bryony plant, is suggested for soreness that's worsened by movement. Arnica, derived from the arnica plant, is renowned for reducing muscle pain and inflammation post-exertion.

Eye Fatigue from Screen Use:

First Aid: The 20-20-20 rule encourages breaks to focus on objects 20 feet away for 20 seconds every 20 minutes. Adjusting the screen to eye level and using artificial tears can reduce eye strain.

Homeopathic: Ruta graveolens, made from the common rue plant, is believed to support eye health and relieve eyestrain associated with reading or screen time.

Motion-Related Vertigo:

First Aid: Sit or lie down to prevent falls. Ginger supplements, acupressure wristbands, or ginger tea might help alleviate symptoms.

Homeopathic: Cocculus indicus, derived from the Indian cockle, is indicated for dizziness caused by motion sickness or travel.

Peptic Ulcers:

First Aid: Avoiding caffeine, spicy foods, and tobacco is advised. Antacids provide short-term relief. Mastic gum and honey have been studied for potential ulcer-soothing effects.

Homeopathic: Arsenicum album, made from arsenic trioxide, might be used for peptic ulcer symptoms characterized by burning pain and anxiety.

Restlessness or Hyperactivity:

First Aid: Creating a structured routine with calming activities can help manage restlessness. Adequate sleep and physical activity contribute to a balanced lifestyle.

Homeopathic: Tarentula hispanica, derived from a type of wolf spider, is thought to address restlessness and hyperactivity.

Throat Irritation from Coughing:

First Aid: Honey mixed with warm water can soothe the throat. Gargling with salt water can alleviate discomfort. A humidifier in the room can prevent throat dryness.

Homeopathic: Belladonna, made from the deadly nightshade plant, is suggested for sudden onset of intense throat irritation.

Mild Constipation:

First Aid: Dietary fiber from fruits, vegetables, and whole grains aids digestion. Prunes, flaxseeds, and psyllium husk can be natural remedies.

Homeopathic: Nux vomica, prepared from the strychnine tree's seeds, is a common choice for constipation, especially when accompanied by frequent, ineffective urges.

Acid Reflux (Heartburn):

First Aid: Elevating the head of the bed prevents stomach acid from flowing back into the esophagus. Licorice root tea might provide soothing effects.

Homeopathic: Pulsatilla, made from windflower, is used for heartburn worsened by consuming rich, fatty foods.

Sudden Tooth Sensitivity

First Aid: Toothpaste designed for sensitive teeth can help alleviate discomfort. Avoiding extremely hot or cold foods can prevent aggravating sensitivity.

Homeopathic: Coffea cruda, derived from unroasted coffee beans, is suggested for sudden, sharp tooth pain.

Minor Sleep Disturbances (Insomnia):

First Aid: Creating a bedtime routine and practicing relaxation techniques, such as meditation or deep breathing, can promote better sleep.

Homeopathic: Coffea cruda is recommended for individuals with an overactive mind interfering with their ability to fall asleep.

Acne Breakouts:

First Aid: Gentle cleansing with salicylic acid or benzoyl peroxide products can help control acne. Using non-comedogenic moisturizers prevents clogged pores.

Homeopathic: Hepar sulphuris, derived from calcium sulfide, might be used for acne with pus-filled eruptions and sensitivity to touch.

Irritation from Inhaled Irritants:

First Aid: Saline nasal irrigation helps flush irritants from the nasal passages. Wearing a mask can protect you from pollutants.

Homeopathic: Ipecacuanha, derived from ipecac root, has been used to alleviate irritation caused by inhaled substances.

Morning Sickness during Pregnancy:

First Aid: Ginger tea or ginger candies can help ease nausea. Snacking on crackers before getting out of bed can also help.

Homeopathic: Sepia, prepared from the ink of the common cuttlefish, might be used for morning sickness accompanied by an aversion to food.

Joint Stiffness from Rheumatoid Arthritis:

First Aid: Applying hot or cold packs can temporarily relieve stiffness. Regular low-impact exercise like swimming can maintain joint flexibility.

Homeopathic: Bryonia and Rhus toxicodendron (Rhus Tox) are common choices for joint issues in homeopathy, each addressing different aspects of discomfort.

Dry Skin:

First Aid: Using a humidifier in dry environments helps maintain skin moisture. Aloe vera gel can provide soothing relief.

Homeopathic: Graphites, derived from graphite minerals, might be chosen for persistent dry skin.

Minor Joint Sprain:

First Aid: Applying a compression bandage can reduce swelling. Gentle range-of-motion exercises aid in preventing stiffness during recovery.

Homeopathic: Ruta graveolens, prepared from the rue plant, is indicated for injuries involving ligaments and tendons.

Dry Skin:

First Aid: Using fragrance-free moisturizers containing ingredients like ceramides and hyaluronic acid can effectively lock in moisture. Avoiding harsh soaps and opting for gentle cleansers is key.

Homeopathic: Graphites, derived from graphite mineral, are often chosen for dry skin that is prone to cracking, oozing, and itching.

Joint Sprain:

First Aid: In addition to R.I.C.E. (Rest, Ice, Compression, Elevation), over-the-counter pain relievers like ibuprofen can help reduce pain and inflammation.

Homeopathic: Ruta graveolens, prepared from the rue plant, is believed to support the healing of ligaments and tendons after a sprain.

Allergic Reactions to Plants:

First Aid: Avoiding scratching is crucial to prevent secondary infections. Applying calamine lotion or aloe vera gel can provide soothing relief.

Homeopathic: Rhus toxicodendron, made from poison ivy, can address allergic reactions that manifest as itchy, blistering rashes.

Head Injury (without loss of consciousness):

First Aid: Even in mild head injuries, closely monitor for symptoms like persistent headache, dizziness, nausea, or changes in behavior.

Homeopathic: Natrum sulphuricum, derived from sodium sulfate, is sometimes used for lingering symptoms after a head injury, especially if they involve headaches or emotional changes.

Hemorrhoids (Piles):

First Aid: Sitz baths, where the lower body is soaked in warm water, can provide relief. Over-the-counter hemorrhoid creams or pads containing witch hazel might help reduce discomfort.

Homeopathic: Aesculus hippocastanum, made from horse chestnut, can address hemorrhoids with pain that radiates to the lower back.

Allergic Reactions to Latex:

First Aid: To prevent future reactions, identify and replace latex-containing products in your environment with hypoallergenic alternatives.

Homeopathic: Apis mellifica, derived from honeybees, may be chosen for mild allergic reactions to latex that involve itching, redness, and swelling.

Bacterial Conjunctivitis (Pink Eye):

First Aid: Frequent hand washing and avoiding touching the eyes can prevent the spread of bacterial conjunctivitis. Over-the-counter lubricating eye drops can alleviate dryness.

Homeopathic: Euphrasia, prepared from the eyebright plant, is believed to address pink eye symptoms like watery discharge and eye irritation.

Hangover:

First Aid: Replenishing electrolytes with sports drinks or oral rehydration solutions can alleviate dehydration. Consuming foods rich in potassium, like bananas, can also help.

Homeopathic: Nux vomica, derived from the strychnine tree's seeds, is often considered for hangover relief, especially when there's headache, nausea, and sensitivity to light and noise.

Flatulence (Gas):

First Aid: Incorporating probiotic-rich foods, like yogurt, can help maintain a healthy gut flora and reduce gas production. Peppermint tea might also offer relief.

Homeopathic: Carbo vegetabilis, prepared from vegetable charcoal, may be indicated for flatulence with bloating and discomfort.

Foot Blisters:

First Aid: Applying antibiotic ointment and covering the blister with a sterile dressing helps prevent infection. Avoiding tight shoes and friction-causing activities is crucial during healing.

Homeopathic: Cantharis, derived from Spanish fly, may help blister healing, particularly when there's a burning sensation.

Stomach Bloating:

First Aid: Consuming foods rich in soluble fiber, like oats and legumes, can promote regular bowel movements and reduce bloating.

Homeopathic: Lycopodium, made from club moss, may be chosen for bloating and indigestion with a sensation of fullness and gas.

Overexertion or Fatigue:

First Aid: Hydrating with electrolyte-rich beverages and consuming complex carbohydrates, like whole grains, can aid in recovery.

Homeopathic: Arnica montana, derived from the arnica plant, is known for its potential to alleviate fatigue resulting from physical strain.

Cough:

First Aid: Consuming honey and warm herbal teas, like chamomile or thyme tea, can help soothe a cough. Steam inhalation with eucalyptus oil can also provide relief.

Homeopathic: Drosera, made from the sundew plant, might be indicated for dry, spasmodic coughs with tickling sensations in the throat.

Gastric Upset from Spicy Foods:

First Aid: Incorporating bland foods like rice, bananas, and applesauce into your diet can help calm the stomach. Ginger tea might offer relief from indigestion.

Homeopathic: Arsenicum album, derived from arsenic trioxide, is often considered for stomach upset with burning pains and restlessness.

Motion-Related Vertigo:

First Aid: When experiencing motion-related vertigo, sitting or lying down helps prevent falls. Avoiding sudden head movements minimizes dizziness. Focusing on a stationary object or the horizon can stabilize your perception.

Homeopathic: Cocculus indicus is well-regarded for motion sickness and travel-induced vertigo. It's believed to ease symptoms like nausea, dizziness, and imbalance. Traveling in cars, boats, or planes can trigger this condition.

Peptic Ulcers:

• First Aid: Peptic ulcers are often caused by the erosion of the stomach lining due to stomach acid. Avoiding spicy and acidic foods, alcohol, and caffeine can mitigate symptoms. Over-the-counter antacids neutralize excess stomach acid and provide relief. A bland diet consisting of easily digestible foods can promote healing.

• Homeopathic: Arsenicum album, with its focus on burning pains, is utilized to address peptic ulcer symptoms. This remedy may be suitable for those who experience burning stomach pain relieved by warmth and drinking warm liquids.

Restlessness or Hyperactivity:

• First Aid: Restlessness and hyperactivity can stem from various factors, including excess energy or underlying conditions. Engaging in calming activities such as reading, deep breathing, or gentle stretching can provide relief. Establishing a consistent daily routine and ensuring sufficient sleep is vital for managing hyperactivity.

• Homeopathic: Tarentula hispanica, derived from the Spanish spider, is thought to aid in restlessness, particularly in children. This remedy could be considered when symptoms include excessive movement, fidgeting, and a need for constant stimulation.

Throat Irritation from Coughing:

• First Aid: Throat irritation from frequent coughing can be eased by staying hydrated to keep the throat moist. Using lozenges containing soothing ingredients like honey or menthol provides temporary relief. Warm liquids such as herbal teas or broths help soothe the throat's lining.

• Homeopathic: Belladonna, known for its affinity for sudden and intense symptoms, may be appropriate for throat irritation with inflammation. It might be considered when symptoms appear rapidly, accompanied by a dry, hot throat and difficulty swallowing.

Constipation:

• First Aid: Mild constipation can result from factors like insufficient fiber intake, dehydration, or lack of physical activity. Drinking plenty of water and consuming fiber-rich foods like fruits, vegetables, and whole grains promote regular bowel movements. Engaging in regular exercise supports digestive health.

• Homeopathic: Nux vomica is often chosen for constipation with a sense of ineffectual urging to pass stool. This remedy might be suitable for individuals who experience a constant desire to have a bowel movement without satisfactory results.

Acid Reflux (Heartburn):

• First Aid: Heartburn, caused by stomach acid flowing back into the esophagus, can be managed by avoiding trigger foods, elevating the head of the bed, and wearing loose-fitting clothing. Over-the-counter antacids neutralize stomach acid, providing relief from discomfort.

• Homeopathic: Pulsatilla, with its emphasis on changeable symptoms, might be relevant for heartburn that worsens after consuming rich, fatty foods. It's often suited for individuals with a mild and yielding disposition.

Sudden Tooth Sensitivity:

• First Aid: Tooth sensitivity can arise from enamel erosion or gum recession. Using toothpaste designed for sensitive teeth containing ingredients like potassium nitrate or stannous fluoride can help alleviate discomfort. Visiting a dentist for an evaluation is important to rule out underlying issues.

• Homeopathic: Coffea cruda, made from coffee beans, is associated with hypersensitivity and throbbing pain. This remedy might be considered when sudden tooth sensitivity is accompanied by an intense sensation of pain.

Sleep Disturbances (Insomnia):

• First Aid: Insomnia can result from stress, anxiety, or disruptions in sleep routine. Practicing relaxation techniques such as meditation or deep breathing before bed promotes better sleep. Maintaining a consistent sleep schedule and creating a calming sleep environment contribute to improved sleep quality.

• Homeopathic: Coffea cruda, prepared from raw coffee beans, might aid in insomnia triggered by an overactive mind. Individuals who experience racing thoughts and mental restlessness might find relief from this remedy.

Overexertion or Fatigue:

First Aid: Rest is crucial to allow the body to recover from overexertion. Prioritize adequate sleep to restore energy levels. Hydration plays a key role in preventing fatigue, so drink water throughout the day. Engage in relaxation techniques like deep breathing or meditation to calm the nervous system.

Homeopathic: Arnica montana, renowned as a remedy for bruising and physical strain, can be beneficial for fatigue resulting from excessive physical activity. Its application extends to sore muscles and general exhaustion.

Mild Cough:

First Aid: Maintaining proper hydration is essential to prevent a dry throat and ease coughing. Using a humidifier adds moisture to the air, reducing throat irritation. Warm liquids soothe the throat, and lozenges containing menthol or honey provide temporary relief.

Homeopathic: Drosera, derived from the sundew plant, is indicated for dry, spasmodic coughs often accompanied by a tickling sensation. It's associated with intense bouts of coughing, particularly worse at night.

Gastric Upset from Spicy Foods:

First Aid: To ease gastric discomfort, avoiding spicy foods temporarily minimizes irritation. Milk can neutralize the heat from spices, and over-the-counter antacids help alleviate acidity. As symptoms subside, reintroduce spicy foods gradually.

Homeopathic: Arsenicum album, used for a range of symptoms, is indicated for gastric upset from highly seasoned or spicy foods. This remedy might be beneficial when accompanied by restlessness and anxiety.

Mild Sinus Headache:

First Aid: Inhaling steam helps alleviate sinus pressure and ease congestion. Applying warm compresses to the forehead can offer relief. Staying hydrated by drinking fluids supports mucus thinning and drainage.

Homeopathic: Belladonna is considered for sinus headaches accompanied by throbbing, intense pain. This remedy is most suitable when symptoms arise suddenly and are aggravated by light, noise, or movement.

Mildew or Mold Irritation:

First Aid: When exposed to mildew or mold, limiting contact with the affected area is vital. Using a mask protects against inhalation of spores. Ventilating the space reduces the concentration of mold. Individuals with mold sensitivity should consult a medical professional.

Homeopathic: Natrum sulphuricum, often chosen for damp conditions, can be relevant for mild irritation resulting from mold exposure. It's indicated when symptoms include nasal discharge and respiratory discomfort.

Urinary Tract Irritation (e.g., from holding urine too long):

First Aid: Frequent emptying of the bladder prevents irritation caused by holding urine for extended periods. Drinking sufficient water maintains urinary health. Avoiding caffeine and acidic foods reduces irritation. Bladder training involves gradually extending the time between bathroom visits.

Homeopathic: Cantharis, known for its affinity for urinary issues, can be considered for burning sensations and discomfort during urination. It's particularly suitable when the urge to urinate is strong and accompanied by pain.

Menstrual Cramps:

First Aid: Applying a heating pad to the abdomen helps relax uterine muscles and ease cramps. Over-the-counter pain relievers provide relief from discomfort. Resting and practicing relaxation techniques contribute to managing menstrual cramps.

Homeopathic: Magnesia phosphorica, indicated for spasmodic pains, can be chosen for menstrual cramps characterized by sharp, shooting pains. This remedy is also used for alleviating muscle cramps.

Sun Sensitivity (Photodermatitis):

First Aid: To prevent photodermatitis, avoid sun exposure during peak hours and wear protective clothing, including sunglasses and wide-brimmed hats. High SPF sunscreen provides a barrier against UV rays.

Homeopathic: Bellis perennis, also known as the daisy, is utilized for sun-sensitive skin reactions. It might be suitable for soothing skin irritation and inflammation caused by sun exposure.

Chafing or Skin Irritation:

First Aid: To prevent chafing, keeping the affected area dry and applying petroleum jelly or aloe vera gel reduces friction. Wearing breathable fabrics can also help prevent further irritation.

Homeopathic: Graphites, derived from graphite, are indicated for skin issues including chafing and eczema. This remedy may be helpful for soothing irritated skin.

Sinus Congestion:

First Aid: Clearing nasal passages with a saline nasal spray provides relief from congestion. Drinking fluids thins mucus and promotes drainage. Inhaling steam eases sinus pressure and aids in mucus clearance.

Homeopathic: Kali bichromicum is indicated for thick, stringy nasal discharge and sinus pressure. It can be considered for sinus congestion with tough, adhesive mucus.

Tennis/Golfer's Elbow:

• First Aid: Resting the affected arm prevents further strain. Applying ice packs to the area reduces inflammation. Over-the-counter pain relievers offer temporary relief.

• Homeopathic: Ruta graveolens, known for its affinity for ligaments and tendons, can be considered for elbow pain resulting from overuse and repetitive strain.

Seasonal Allergies:

• First Aid: Managing seasonal allergies involves staying indoors during peak pollen times, using air purifiers, and rinsing nasal passages with saline solution. These measures reduce exposure to allergens.

• Homeopathic: Euphrasia, prepared from the eyebright plant, is chosen for eye irritation and nasal discharge associated with allergies. It can be suitable for alleviating allergy-related symptoms.

Mild Allergic Reactions to Topical Substances (e.g., rashes from cosmetics):

• First Aid: Ceasing the use of the product causing the allergic reaction is essential. Washing the affected area helps remove any residue. Applying a mild hydrocortisone cream reduces inflammation and itching.

- Homeopathic: Graphites, derived from carbon, can be considered for skin rashes and eczema resulting from allergic reactions. This remedy may offer relief from skin irritation and promote healing.

Tendonitis or Overuse Injury:

First Aid: Resting the affected area allows for recovery. Applying ice packs helps reduce inflammation. Using a compression bandage or brace provides support to the injured area.

Homeopathic: Ruta graveolens, indicated for injuries to tendons and ligaments, can be chosen for tendonitis and overuse injuries. This remedy may aid in promoting healing and reducing discomfort.

Cuts and Scrapes on the Tongue (e.g., biting tongue accidentally):

First Aid: Gargling with warm saltwater helps cleanse the affected area. Avoiding hot and spicy foods prevents further irritation. Applying a soothing gel or ointment provides relief and supports healing.

Homeopathic: Nitricum Acidum, prepared from nitric acid, can be considered for healing cuts and scrapes on the tongue. This remedy might help alleviate discomfort and promote recovery.

Overactive Bladder (Urinary Urgency):

First Aid: Managing an overactive bladder involves limiting caffeine and alcohol intake, practicing bladder training to gradually extend the time between bathroom visits, and doing Kegel exercises to strengthen pelvic muscles.

Homeopathic: Causticum, indicated for urinary issues, can be chosen for urinary urgency and involuntary urination. This remedy may assist in managing these symptoms.

Restlessness from Teething (in infants):

First Aid: Providing teething toys or a cold washcloth for infants to chew on offers relief. Offering comfort and cuddling can soothe restlessness during the teething process.

Homeopathic: Chamomilla, derived from chamomile, is indicated for teething restlessness and irritability in infants. This remedy can provide comfort during this challenging phase.

Asthma Symptoms:

First Aid: For individuals with asthma, using prescribed inhalers as needed is essential. Identifying and avoiding triggers helps prevent asthma symptoms. Seeking medical attention is crucial if symptoms worsen.

Homeopathic: Natrum sulphuricum, chosen for damp-related symptoms, can be considered for asthma symptoms aggravated by damp weather. This remedy might offer support in managing respiratory discomfort.

Allergic Reactions to Animal Dander:

First Aid: Limiting exposure to pets, using air purifiers, and washing hands after touching animals reduces the risk of allergic reactions to animal dander.

Homeopathic: Arsenicum album, known for its affinity for allergies, can be considered for mild allergic reactions to animal dander. This remedy may assist in managing symptoms.

Leg Cramps (e.g., nocturnal cramps):

First Aid: Gently stretching and massaging the affected muscles helps alleviate leg cramps. Using warm compresses or taking a warm bath can relax the muscles and provide relief.

Homeopathic: Magnesia phosphorica, chosen for spasmodic pains, can aid in alleviating leg cramps and spasms. This remedy is particularly relevant for cramps that are relieved by warmth.

Indigestion from overeating:

First Aid: Eating smaller portions and avoiding lying down immediately after meals helps prevent indigestion. Taking a short walk after eating promotes digestion. Practicing moderation in food intake is key to preventing discomfort.

Homeopathic: Nux vomica, derived from the poison nut, can help with indigestion caused by overeating and consuming spicy foods. This remedy may assist in relieving digestive discomfort.

Sudden Anxiety or Nervousness:

First Aid: Managing sudden anxiety involves practicing deep breathing and relaxation techniques. Seeking support from a friend or family member can provide solace.

Asthma Symptoms:

• First Aid: Mild asthma symptoms can be managed with a combination of preventive measures and appropriate medication. If prescribed, using an inhaler as directed can help open the airways and relieve symptoms. Avoiding triggers such as allergens, smoke, and cold air is important to prevent exacerbation. Maintaining a clean and dust-free living environment, using air purifiers, and covering bedding can reduce exposure to allergens.

• Homeopathic: Natrum sulphuricum, made from sulfate of sodium, is indicated for asthma symptoms that worsen in damp weather. It can help address breathing difficulties and wheezing associated with mild asthma.

Allergic Reactions to Animal Dander:

• First Aid: Managing minor allergic reactions to animal dander involves reducing exposure to the allergen. Limiting contact with pets, using air purifiers to filter out dander, and washing hands and clothes after interacting with animals can help minimize symptoms. Regularly cleaning and vacuuming living spaces can also reduce dander buildup.

• Homeopathic: Arsenicum album, prepared from arsenic trioxide, can provide relief from mild allergic reactions to animal dander. It addresses symptoms like sneezing, runny nose, and skin itching.

Leg Cramps (e.g., nocturnal cramps):

• First Aid: Preventing and alleviating mild leg cramps involves gentle stretching and massaging of the affected muscles. Staying hydrated and maintaining a balanced diet rich in electrolytes can help prevent muscle cramps. Applying warm compresses or taking a warm bath can also provide relief.

• Homeopathic: Magnesia phosphorica, prepared from magnesium phosphate, is known to alleviate muscle cramps and spasms. It can help relax muscles and ease discomfort.

Indigestion from overeating:

• First Aid: Mild indigestion from overeating can be managed by adopting healthy eating habits. Consuming smaller portions and avoiding heavy, fatty, and spicy foods can prevent discomfort. Taking a short walk after meals can aid digestion by promoting gentle movement in the digestive tract.

• Homeopathic: Nux vomica, derived from the strychnine tree's seeds, is indicated for indigestion caused by overeating and excessive consumption of rich foods. It can help address symptoms like bloating, flatulence, and irritability.

Sudden Anxiety or Nervousness:

• First Aid: Coping with sudden anxiety or nervousness involves practicing relaxation techniques to calm the mind. Deep breathing exercises, mindfulness, and grounding techniques can help manage overwhelming emotions. Seeking support from a friend, family member, or mental health professional can provide reassurance and guidance.

• Homeopathic: Aconitum napellus, derived from the monkshood plant, is used for sudden anxiety, fear, and panic. It can help address acute episodes of nervousness and restlessness.

Dry Eyes:

• First Aid: Mild dry eyes can be relieved by using artificial tears or lubricating eye drops to provide moisture. Taking breaks from prolonged screen time and ensuring proper hydration can also contribute to eye comfort.

• Homeopathic: Euphrasia, also known as eyebright, is used to alleviate dry, irritated eyes. It can help soothe eye discomfort and promote tear production.

Nosebleeds:

- First Aid: Nosebleeds, also known as epistaxis, can be managed effectively by following these steps. Have the person sit upright and lean slightly forward to prevent blood from flowing down the throat. Gently pinch the soft part of the nose just below the nasal bridge for 10-15 minutes. This helps apply pressure to the bleeding vessel and encourages clotting. It's important to avoid tilting the head back, as this can cause blood to flow down the throat and lead to swallowing or choking.

- Homeopathic: Ferrum phosphoricum, made from iron phosphate, is a remedy that can be considered for nosebleeds due to minor injuries. It can help control bleeding and promote healing of the nasal blood vessels.

Burns from Hot Objects (e.g., touching a hot pan):

• First Aid: Mild burns from hot objects can be treated promptly to prevent further injury. Immediately cool the affected area under cold, running water for several minutes. This helps lower the skin temperature and minimize tissue damage. Avoid using ice or icy water, as extreme cold can cause additional damage. After cooling, cover the burn with a sterile non-stick bandage or clean cloth.

• Homeopathic: Cantharis, prepared from the Spanish fly beetle, is used for burns with intense pain, blistering, and burning sensation. It can provide relief from the discomfort associated with minor burns.

Indigestion:

• First Aid: Indigestion, characterized by discomfort or pain in the upper abdomen, can often be managed through dietary adjustments and lifestyle changes. Avoid heavy, fatty, and spicy foods that can exacerbate symptoms. Opt for smaller, more frequent meals and avoid lying down immediately after eating. Consuming ginger or peppermint tea can aid digestion and soothe the stomach.

• Homeopathic: Carbo vegetabilis, derived from vegetable charcoal, is indicated for bloating and flatulence. It can provide relief from indigestion and discomfort caused by gas accumulation in the digestive tract.

Mild Heat Exhaustion:

• First Aid: Heat exhaustion can occur when the body loses too much water and salt due to excessive heat and sweating. Move the person to a cooler area, such as an air-conditioned room or shade. Encourage them to drink cool water or an electrolyte-rich beverage to rehydrate. Loosen tight clothing and use cool compresses to lower body temperature.

• Homeopathic: Gelsemium, derived from the yellow jasmine plant, is used for weakness and fatigue associated with heat exhaustion. It can help alleviate symptoms and support recovery.

Gastrointestinal Upset (e.g., traveler's diarrhea):

• First Aid: Traveler's diarrhea, often caused by consuming contaminated food or water, can lead to discomfort and dehydration. Stay hydrated by drinking oral rehydration solutions to replenish lost fluids and electrolytes. Avoid consuming spicy, greasy, and raw foods until symptoms subside. Rest and allow your body time to recover.

• Homeopathic: Arsenicum album, prepared from arsenic trioxide, is indicated for diarrhea accompanied by weakness, restlessness, and anxiety. It can aid in alleviating symptoms and promoting recovery.

Emotional Shock or Trauma:

• First Aid: Experiencing emotional shock or trauma can be distressing. Offer comfort and support by listening attentively and providing a safe space for the individual to express their feelings. Encourage deep breathing exercises to help calm the nervous system. If the emotional distress persists, consider seeking professional help from a therapist or counselor.

• Homeopathic: Ignatia derived from the St. Ignatius bean, is used for emotional distress, grief, and shock. It can help address acute emotional reactions and provide relief during challenging times.

Also, aconite is useful

Dehydration:

• First Aid: Dehydration occurs when the body loses more fluids than it takes in. Drink plenty of fluids, particularly water or oral rehydration solutions, to restore hydration levels. Aim to consume fluids throughout the day, even if you're not feeling thirsty. Avoid caffeinated and alcoholic beverages, as they can contribute to dehydration.

• Homeopathic: Veratrum album, prepared from white hellebore, is indicated for profuse, watery diarrhea leading to dehydration. It can help address symptoms of fluid loss and support rehydration.

Remember that while first aid measures and homeopathic remedies can be helpful for minor situations, professional medical advice should be sought for severe or persistent symptoms. Homeopathic remedies should be used under the guidance of a qualified practitioner, especially if you have any underlying health conditions or are taking other medications.

Heat exhaustion

- First Aid: Heat exhaustion can occur when the body loses too much water and salt due to excessive heat and sweating. Move the person to a cooler area, such as an air-conditioned room or shade. Encourage them to drink cool water or an electrolyte-rich beverage to rehydrate. Loosen tight clothing and use cool compresses to lower body temperature.

- Homeopathic: Gelsemium, derived from the yellow jasmine plant, is used for weakness and fatigue associated with heat exhaustion. It can help alleviate symptoms and support recovery.

Gastrointestinal Upset (e.g., traveler's diarrhea):

- First Aid: Traveler's diarrhea, often caused by consuming contaminated food or water, can lead to discomfort and dehydration. Stay hydrated by drinking oral rehydration solutions to replenish lost fluids and electrolytes. Avoid consuming spicy, greasy, and raw foods until symptoms subside. Rest and allow your body time to recover.

- Homeopathic: Arsenicum album, prepared from arsenic trioxide, is indicated for diarrhea accompanied by weakness, restlessness, and anxiety. It can aid in alleviating symptoms and promoting recovery.

Plantar Fasciitis (Heel Pain):
   - First Aid: Rest the foot, apply ice packs, and use supportive footwear with cushioned insoles to alleviate the discomfort. It's essential to avoid activities that worsen the pain and allow the inflamed plantar fascia to heal properly.
   - Homeopathic: Rhus toxicodendron is a remedy known for assisting with plantar fasciitis-related heel pain. It can help reduce inflammation and provide relief from the stabbing sensation that often accompanies this condition.
   Wrist Tendinitis (e.g., from repetitive movements):
   - First Aid: Address wrist tendinitis by giving the affected wrist ample rest, applying ice packs to reduce inflammation, and considering wrist splints for added support during daily activities. Avoiding repetitive movements that exacerbate the pain is crucial for a swift recovery.
   - Homeopathic: Ruta graveolens is a remedy that can be beneficial for addressing wrist tendinitis and repetitive strain injuries. It assists in alleviating pain, stiffness, and discomfort in the wrist area.
   Acid Indigestion from Stress (Nervous Dyspepsia):
   - First Aid: Stress-induced acid indigestion can be managed by avoiding acidic foods and beverages. Opt for water or milk to soothe the discomfort. Over-the-counter antacids can provide relief. Managing stress through relaxation techniques is crucial to prevent recurring symptoms.
   - Homeopathic: Arsenicum album is a remedy that addresses acid indigestion triggered by stress. It helps ease symptoms like

burning sensations and discomfort, especially when stress plays a significant role.

Diarrhea from Traveler's Tummy:

- First Aid: Mild diarrhea from travel-related causes can be managed by staying hydrated

and using oral rehydration solutions to replace lost electrolytes. It's important to consume easily digestible foods, like rice, bananas, and toast, and to avoid dairy, caffeine, and alcohol until recovery.

- Homeopathic: Podophyllum is often recommended for diarrhea that is profuse and gushing, which may be accompanied by abdominal cramping and discomfort. It can be considered when the symptoms match this specific profile.

Motion Sickness:

- First Aid: Motion sickness can be addressed by focusing on the horizon or closing one's eyes to reduce the sensory conflict that causes nausea. Fresh air can also alleviate symptoms, so it's helpful to step outside if possible or use air conditioning in a vehicle. Over-the-counter motion sickness medications may be useful for preventing and treating symptoms.

- Homeopathic: Cocculus indicus is commonly used for the relief of motion sickness, especially when there is a feeling of dizziness and nausea with an inability to endure the sight or smell of food.

Bruising:

- First Aid: To manage minor bruising, apply a cold compress immediately to reduce swelling and help numb the pain. Elevate the affected area if possible to minimize blood flow, which can help reduce the size of the bruise.

- Homeopathic: Arnica montana is a popular remedy for bruises and is believed to help reduce swelling and decrease pain, speeding up the healing process.

Sunburn:

- First Aid: For mild sunburn, it is important to cool the skin by applying cool compresses or taking a cool bath. Moisturizing lotions that contain aloe vera can soothe the affected skin. Stay hydrated and avoid further sun exposure while the burn heals.

- Homeopathic: Belladonna is often recommended for sunburn when the skin is hot, red, and burning.

Dry Cough:

- First Aid: Soothe a mild dry cough by staying hydrated to keep the throat moist. A humidifier can provide relief by adding moisture to the air. Warm liquids and lozenges can also alleviate discomfort and reduce coughing episodes.

- Homeopathic: Drosera is a remedy that offers relief from dry, spasmodic coughs. It addresses the irritation in the throat that triggers bouts of coughing.

Oral Thrush (Mouth Fungus):

- First Aid: Practicing good oral hygiene is key to managing mild oral thrush. Use antifungal mouthwashes as directed and avoid sugary foods that can worsen the condition. Maintaining a clean mouth and preventing overgrowth of the fungus is essential.

- Homeopathic: Borax is a remedy that aids in thrush with painful, sensitive gums. It can help alleviate discomfort and promote healing in the affected areas.

Dizziness from Inner Ear Issues:

- First Aid: Managing mild dizziness due to inner ear issues involves sitting or lying down to prevent falls, avoiding sudden head movements that worsen the dizziness, and performing vestibular exercises to improve balance.

- Homeopathic: Conium maculatum is a remedy known for addressing dizziness arising from inner ear problems. It supports the body's efforts to restore equilibrium and alleviate the sensation of spinning.

Restlessness from Stress or Anxiety:

- First Aid: Coping with restlessness caused by stress or anxiety involves practicing deep breathing, engaging in calming activities like meditation, and seeking support from friends or family. Stress management techniques can significantly reduce feelings of restlessness.

- Homeopathic: Coffea cruda is a remedy that assists with restlessness and sleeplessness due to mental agitation. It can help calm the mind and promote relaxation.

Shoulder Impingement (Rotator Cuff Tendinitis):

- First Aid: Ease mild shoulder impingement pain by resting the affected shoulder, applying ice packs to reduce inflammation, and performing gentle shoulder stretches to maintain flexibility. Avoiding activities that strain the shoulder is essential for recovery.

- Homeopathic: Rhus Toxicodendron is a remedy that can be beneficial for shoulder impingement pain. It helps reduce pain, inflammation, and stiffness associated with this condition.

Tension Headache:

- First Aid: Alleviating mild tension headaches involves practicing relaxation techniques, such as deep breathing or meditation. Applying a warm compress to the forehead and resting in a quiet, dimly lit room can provide relief.

- Homeopathic: Gelsemium is a remedy that addresses tension headaches caused by stress and fatigue. It helps ease the dull, heavy sensation often associated with these headaches.

Urinary Tract Infection (UTI):

- First Aid: Managing a mild UTI includes staying hydrated with water, avoiding caffeine and alcohol that can irritate the bladder, and using over-the-counter pain relievers to alleviate discomfort. Seeking medical attention if symptoms persist is essential.

- Homeopathic: Cantharis is a remedy that can assist with UTI symptoms, including the burning sensation during urination and frequent urges to urinate.

Temporomandibular Joint (TMJ) Discomfort:

- First Aid: Addressing minor TMJ discomfort involves avoiding chewing tough foods that strain the jaw, applying warm compresses to relax the jaw muscles, and practicing gentle jaw exercises to improve flexibility and alleviate tension.

- Homeopathic: Hypericum is a remedy that can help with gum irritation and pain. It supports healing and provides relief from discomfort caused by orthodontic appliances.

Canker Sores (Aphthous Ulcers):

- First Aid: Managing minor canker sores includes avoiding acidic and spicy foods that can irritate the sores. Over-the-counter oral gels can provide relief, and maintaining good oral hygiene helps prevent infection and promote healing.

- Homeopathic: Borax is a remedy that aids in canker sores with painful ulcers. It assists in reducing pain and promoting the healing process.

Restlessness from Skin Irritation (e.g., from rashes or insect bites):

- First Aid: Soothe restlessness caused by skin irritations with calamine lotion. Avoid scratching to prevent worsening the irritation. Keeping the affected area clean and dry supports healing.

- Homeopathic: Apis mellifica is a remedy that helps address restlessness and itching from skin irritations, relieving discomfort and promoting healing.

Snoring (Infrequent and non-obstructive):

- First Aid: To manage minor snoring, sleeping on your side can help prevent the airway collapse that contributes to snoring. Nasal strips can help improve nasal airflow, and avoiding alcohol before bedtime can reduce muscle relaxation that exacerbates snoring.

- Homeopathic: Nux vomica is a remedy that can assist with snoring caused by overindulgence. It supports the body in maintaining healthy sleep patterns and reducing snoring episodes.

Restlessness from Teething (in toddlers):

- First Aid: Comforting a restless toddler during teething involves providing teething toys or a cold washcloth to chew on. Offering soothing measures like cuddling and offering cool, non-solid foods can provide relief from discomfort.

- Homeopathic: Chamomilla is a remedy that can be used for restlessness and irritability during teething. It supports the child's comfort and helps ease the symptoms associated with teething.

Shoulder Impingement (Rotator Cuff Tendinitis)

- First Aid: To manage shoulder impingement pain, rest is crucial to allow the injured tissues to heal. Applying ice packs in the initial stages can help reduce inflammation. Gentle shoulder stretches can improve flexibility and promote healing.

- Homeopathic: Bryonia is a remedy that can aid in arthritis-related stiffness and pain. It helps alleviate discomfort and supports the body in addressing inflammation associated with joint problems.

Muscle Soreness after Exercise

- First Aid: After exercise-induced muscle soreness, gentle stretching exercises can promote blood flow and alleviate stiffness. Applying a warm compress can also help relax muscles and reduce discomfort.

- Homeopathic: Ruta graveolens is a remedy that aids muscle soreness and stiffness after exercise. It supports the body's natural healing process and helps relieve post-workout discomfort and arnica.

Stiff Neck or Neck Strain:

- First Aid: For minor stiff neck or neck strain, applying a warm compress can help relax tense muscles. Gentle neck stretches and avoiding straining the neck during activities can promote recovery.

- Homeopathic: Ruta graveolens is a remedy that helps with neck stiffness and pain. It addresses discomfort caused by muscle strain and supports the neck's flexibility.

Car Motion Sickness:

- First Aid: To manage car motion sickness, sitting in the front seat and focusing on the horizon can reduce feelings of nausea. Avoiding activities exacerbating symptoms, such as reading or using electronic devices, can help prevent discomfort.

- Homeopathic: Cocculus indicus is a remedy that can help with car motion sickness and dizziness. It supports the body in overcoming the sensation of motion-related nausea.

If you wish to pursue further information and perhaps certification or training in first aid methodology, the following organizations listed may benefit you.

American Red Cross: A humanitarian organization that provides emergency assistance, disaster relief, and education. They offer first aid, CPR, and AED training courses.

American Heart Association: A nonprofit organization that promotes cardiovascular health and provides training in CPR, first aid, and advanced cardiac life support.

YMCA: A community organization that offers a variety of programs, including first aid and CPR training, swimming and water safety courses, and health and fitness programs.

National Safety Council: A nonprofit organization promoting safety and preventing injuries in workplaces, homes, and communities. They offer various safety training programs, including first aid and CPR.

St. John Ambulance: A volunteer-led organization that provides first aid training, health and safety courses, and medical services at events to improve public health and safety.

International Red Cross and Red Crescent Movement: A global humanitarian network that offers aid during emergencies, disasters, and conflicts. They provide first aid training and disaster response services.

Wilderness Medical Associates: A company specializing in wilderness medicine education, offering courses on wilderness first aid, advanced life support, and wilderness EMT training.

National CPR Association: An online resource for CPR and first aid certification and training courses, providing flexible options for individuals seeking life-saving skills.

Emergency Care & Safety Institute: An organization offering first aid, CPR, and safety training programs for workplaces, schools, and the community.

American Safety & Health Institute: Provides training programs in first aid, CPR, AED, and various other health and safety topics to individuals and organizations.

Medic First Aid: Offers a range of CPR and first aid training courses, focusing on providing practical skills and knowledge for emergencies.

National Association for Search and Rescue (NASAR): Provides training and resources for search and rescue professionals and volunteers, including wilderness first aid courses.

National Association of Emergency Medical Technicians (NAEMT): Represents emergency medical technicians and offers training and education programs to enhance prehospital care.

American Academy of Orthopaedic Surgeons (AAOS): Provides resources and courses on orthopedic trauma and emergency care for healthcare professionals.

Wilderness Medicine Institute: Offers wilderness medicine courses for outdoor enthusiasts, healthcare professionals, and rescue teams.

National CPR Foundation: Offers online CPR and first aid certification courses that can be completed at the learner's own pace.

Remote Medical International: Provides medical training and services for remote and austere environments, including wilderness first aid and remote medical training.

National Association of Professional First Aiders: Focuses on promoting professional first aid and emergency care standards through education and training.

Life Support Training Institute: Offers ACLS, BLS, PALS, and other life support training courses for healthcare providers.

Emergency Care & Safety Institute (ECSI): Provides comprehensive emergency care training programs for individuals and organizations.

Canadian Red Cross: Offers first aid and CPR training, disaster response, and humanitarian assistance in Canada.

Australian Red Cross: Provides disaster relief, blood donation, and community services in Australia, including first aid and CPR training.

British Red Cross: Delivers first aid training, health and social care, and humanitarian services in the United Kingdom.

Irish Red Cross: Offers first aid and health and safety training, along with humanitarian services in Ireland.

New Zealand Red Cross: Provides first aid training, disaster response, and community services in New Zealand.

Canadian Lifesaving Society: Focuses on water safety education and training, including first aid, lifeguarding, and water rescue.

Royal Life Saving Society (UK): Promotes water safety and provides training in lifesaving, first aid, and water rescue in the United Kingdom.

These organizations are vital in educating individuals and communities about first aid, safety, and emergency response, ultimately contributing to safer and healthier societies.

Conclusion to the chapter on homeopathic first aid:

This chapter has presented a captivating array of first aid situations where homeopathic medicine showcases its remarkable efficacy. The scenarios explored here offer a mere glimpse into the vast potential of homeopathy. From minor injuries to discomforts and from restlessness to specific conditions, each homeopathic remedy brings a unique resonance with the body's inherent healing mechanisms.

Yet, it's important to emphasize that the scope of homeopathic medicine extends far beyond the boundaries of this chapter. The potential applications are as diverse as the human experience itself. The exploration of homeopathy doesn't end here; it is an open invitation to embark on a journey of deeper understanding and discovery.

Integrating homeopathy into conventional healthcare practices has shown promise as an adjunctive approach. Its holistic nature aligns with treating the symptoms and addressing the underlying imbalances contributing to our ailments. By embracing homeopathic remedies, we tap into the healing wisdom of nature that has been cherished for centuries.

Homeopathy's ability to work harmoniously with the body's healing processes is a testament to its effectiveness. It complements and extends the realm of minor first aid solutions, presenting a natural option that respects the body's innate intelligence. This is particularly important in today's world, where many seek alternatives to synthetic medications and wish to minimize their exposure to unnecessary chemicals.

As you delve into the wealth of information in this chapter, I encourage you to view it as a starting point, an introduction to a holistic approach to well-being. The remedies mentioned here are like keys that can unlock the body's potential to heal itself, offering gentle yet potent support when it's needed the most.

With an open heart and a curious mind, you can explore further and expand your knowledge of homeopathic medicine. Through self-care and the guidance of qualified practitioners, you can embark on a transformative journey toward more excellent health and vitality. By incorporating these remedies into your daily life, you're inviting the power of nature to join hands with your body's healing abilities.

In this journey, you're not alone. Homeopathy has a rich history, a global community of practitioners, and a wealth of literature to guide you. As you embrace this holistic path, may you find empowerment in taking charge of your health and well-being? And as you do, remember that homeopathic medicine is not just a remedy; it's a philosophy that respects the intricate interplay of the body, mind, and spirit.

So, armed with the insights from this chapter, step forward with confidence. Let homeopathy become a source of comfort, a friend who stands by you in times of need. May it encourage you to explore the potential of a more natural, holistic approach to health—one that resonates with the wisdom of ages and the rhythm of nature. As you incorporate homeopathy into your life, may you find balance, harmony, and a renewed sense of vitality.

Chapter 5: The use of astrology in case-taking

This chapter deals with the intriguing approach of using astrology as part of the case-taking process in homeopathic medicine. It discusses how astrology aids practitioners in understanding patient's traits, tendencies, and susceptibilities. By combining homeopathic principles with astrological analysis, practitioners can gain deeper insights into their patient's unique constitutions.

A contemporary fusion of traditional astrological principles with humanistic psychology forms an innovative approach focusing on an individual's inner development, self-awareness, and personal growth. This modern method shifts away from predicting specific events and instead centers on understanding an individual's psyche to catalyze their expansion journey.

The Birth Chart's Role as a Blueprint

Central to this approach is the belief that a birth chart serves as a symbolic blueprint, outlining an individual's potential, psychological inclinations, and life experiences. Instead of predetermined destinies, the philosophy suggests that individuals hold the power to shape their lives through self-awareness and conscious choices.

Practitioners of this approach delve into the psychological dynamics reflected by planetary positions, aspects, and other astrological factors within the birth chart. Viewed as a canvas, the birth chart portrays archetypal energies and symbolic patterns that offer insights into an individual's motivations, strengths, challenges, and growth opportunities.

An intriguing facet of this method lies in incorporating humanistic psychology's insights. Principles from humanistic psychology, such as personal development and the significance of an individual's subjective experience, enhance the interpretation of astrological elements. This integration deepens the understanding of an individual's journey.

This method places significant emphasis on empowerment and self-responsibility. It encourages individuals to actively engage with the insights provided by their birth chart, using them as tools for self-reflection, self-discovery, and personal empowerment. By recognizing the potentials and challenges indicated in the birth chart, individuals can make informed choices that resonate with their authentic selves.

Archetypal Insights and Influences of Carl Jung

Drawing from the concepts of Carl Jung, such as archetypes and the collective unconscious, this approach interprets the birth chart's symbols as representations of universal themes and patterns. This Jungian perspective allows practitioners and individuals to explore profound layers of the human psyche and connect with shared human experiences these archetypes represent.

Practitioners often engage in dialogue and counseling with clients. This interactive process involves guiding individuals in understanding the insights provided by their birth chart. Astrologers assist individuals in identifying their strengths, challenges, and potential life paths, fostering deeper self-awareness and aiding in informed decision-making.

The ultimate aim of this approach is to nurture self-awareness and personal growth. By exploring the birth chart's symbolism, individuals gain insights into their motivations, desires, and potential challenges. This self-knowledge empowers them to make conscious choices, overcome obstacles, and evolve as individuals.

A distinctive aspect of this approach is its emphasis on an individual's capacity to transcend and transform the energies indicated in their birth chart. Instead of being confined by astrological influences, individuals are encouraged to actively engage with and shape their lives according to their aspirations, surpassing limitations and fulfilling their potential.

In summary, this innovative fusion of astrology and humanistic psychology provides a lens through which individuals can delve into themselves, make informed choices, and embark on journeys of personal growth, bridging the gap between cosmic energies and the human experience.

Introduction: Exploring the Harmony of Celestial and Energetic Healing in Homeopathic Practice.

In the vast expanse of medicine, where science meets the mystique of metaphysics, a captivating interplay unfolds between two seemingly diverse realms: astrology and homeopathy. Embarking on this chapter's journey, we illuminate the intricate threads that intricately weave these disciplines together. Through this exploration, a rich tapestry of healing emerges, transcending conventional boundaries of health and wellness.

At the heart of our exploration lies a profound belief: the positions of celestial bodies at birth hold sway over an individual's constitution and life path. Astrology, an age-old art, suggests that these cosmic configurations imprint a unique blueprint on each individual, impacting not only character and destiny but also health predisposition.

Parallel to the cosmic symphony of astrology is homeopathy, a healing art operating on the "like cures like" principle. This philosophy posits that substance evoking symptoms in a healthy person can, when potentized, alleviate similar symptoms in someone ailing. Homeopathic remedies, through meticulous dilution and succession, capture the vibrational essence of natural substances to activate the body's innate healing.

What ties astrology and homeopathy is the belief that cosmic energies, whether from celestial bodies or potentized remedies, influence the human experience. Stellar positions reflect universal energies resonating within an individual's microcosm of body, mind, and spirit. The interplay between these cosmic forces and the body's wisdom forms the bedrock of this convergence.

Astrology's classification into elemental categories

- Fire, Earth, Air, and Water - mirrors homeopathy's understanding of constitutions. Each fundamental type corresponds to distinct personality traits, physical tendencies, and potential health imbalances. Fire types radiate warmth but might battle inflammation; Earth types of ground may face sluggish digestion.

This parallel underscores the intricate dance of celestial and constitutional influences.

As planets traverse the heavens, their transits weave patterns astrologers interpret for insights into life events. Likewise, these cosmic movements can trigger health episodes, particularly in individuals predisposed to certain conditions. A challenging Saturn transit might herald stress and bone-related issues. By integrating these insights with homeopathic remedies, a comprehensive health approach takes shape.

Yet, within these profound insights, ethical considerations arise. While astrology provides invaluable guidance, it's vital to approach health predictions thoughtfully. A holistic perspective harmonizes astrological insights with traditional homeopathic assessment, spotlighting the significance of integrative, balanced care.

In the enchanting union of astrology and homeopathy, a harmonious symphony emerges - one where celestial movements and potentized remedies converge to create a holistic tableau of healing. Join us as we delve into the depths of this intertwined dance, where cosmic energies embrace individual well-being, illuminating pathways of transformation and balance.

Planetary Rulership and Healing Remedies: A Celestial Symphony

Within the intricate interplay of celestial energies and healing practices, a fascinating correspondence emerges between the planets and specific remedies within the realm of homeopathy. This alignment, rooted in archetypal symbolism and shared qualities, unveils a profound connection between the cosmic and the human.

Astrology assigns specific planets to govern different zodiac signs, endowing each world with a unique set of archetypal qualities. Homeopathy, in its exploration of the vibrational essence of substances, similarly categorizes remedies based on the archetypal qualities they encapsulate. This shared archetypal resonance bridges the celestial and the healing realms, where symbolic energies intertwine to influence well-being.

In astrology, planets hold dominion over specific bodily systems and health tendencies. This alignment extends to the world of homeopathy, where remedies attributed to particular planets are believed to resonate with the corresponding physical systems. For instance, Mercury, associated with communication, might find its echo in therapies used to address throat-related issues. This correspondence echoes the ancient belief that our bodies are microcosmic reflections of the universe's macrocosmic patterns.

The planets and some influences on the human body

Mars and Inflammation: The Fiery Healing Force

Mars, the fiery planet, is linked to qualities of action, energy, and sometimes aggression. In homeopathy, Mars' emotional nature resonates with conditions involving inflammation and heat, such as fever or infections. Remedies attributed to Mars are often employed to counteract these inflammatory tendencies, seeking to restore balance within the body. This connection underscores the deep-rooted belief in the resonance between elemental forces and bodily imbalances.

Venus and Harmony: Embracing Balance

Venus, associated with beauty, love, and aesthetics, finds its reflection in homeopathic remedies to harmonize the body. Venusian treatments might be selected to address conditions related to skin health, hormonal imbalances, or emotional well-being. The qualities of balance and harmony attributed to Venus align with the intent of these remedies, promoting a holistic approach to wellness that encompasses physical and emotional realms.

Saturn and Structure: The Foundation of Health

Saturn's role as the taskmaster of the zodiac aligns with its association with structure and discipline. In homeopathy, remedies linked to Saturn are often used to address issues related to bones, joints, and structural integrity. Saturn's archetype reflects the need for maintaining integrity and stability, mirroring the healing intent of these remedies. The interplay between cosmic symbolism and physical well-being underscores the belief that health is intricately tied to the harmonious alignment of energies.

Sun and Vitality: Illuminating the Healing Path

The Sun, symbolic of vitality, consciousness, and life force, corresponds with remedies that restore energy and vibrancy. These remedies might address fatigue, lack of spirit, or disconnection. The Sun's archetype of illumination and life mirrors the healing aim of these remedies, reminding us that healing involves not just the body but also the revitalization of the spirit.

Moon and Emotional Well-being: Nurturing the Soul

The Moon's association with emotions and the subconscious is mirrored in homeopathic remedies focused on emotional well-being. Moon-related treatments might address mood imbalances, emotional sensitivity, or sleep disturbances. The Moon's archetype of reflection and receptivity resonates with the emotional healing these remedies aim to provide. This connection reaffirms that emotions and psyche are integral to overall health.

Mercury and Communication: A Path to Clarity

Mercury's domain of communication, intellect, and versatility finds its parallel in homeopathic remedies used to address conditions involving the nervous system, cognition, or communication issues. Remedies attributed to Mercury might be chosen to support mental clarity, cognitive function, and effective communication. This alignment reinforces the interconnectedness of cognitive well-being with the celestial dance.

Jupiter and Expansion: Nurturing Growth

Jupiter's expansive and benevolent qualities align with remedies to support growth and overall well-being. Therapies attributed to Jupiter might be employed to address issues related to digestion, metabolism, and overall vitality. Jupiter's archetype of growth and abundance resonates with the healing intent of these remedies, encouraging a holistic approach that nurtures physical and spiritual growth.

Uranus, Neptune, and Pluto: Transformational Forces

Modern astrology incorporates the outer planets – Uranus, Neptune, and Pluto – each associated with transformative energies. Similarly, within homeopathy, remedies attributed to these planets might be selected for profound healing shifts or conditions that require a deeper level of transformation. These planetary energies mirror the potential for radical change and evolution within the healing journey.

Symbiosis of Symbols: Cosmic Harmony in Healing

The alignment between planetary symbolism in astrology and the archetypal qualities of homeopathic remedies presents an intricate tapestry where cosmic energies and healing substances intertwine. This symbiotic relationship underscores the ancient belief that the universe's wisdom is imprinted within the microcosm of the human body. As we delve into this interplay between planets and potentized remedies, we uncover a layer of resonance that bridges the celestial and the human, inviting us to consider the profound connection between cosmic energies and the art of healing.

At the heart of the intricate dance between astrology and homeopathy lies a captivating interplay, one where the symbolism of celestial bodies finds resonance with the archetypal qualities of homeopathic remedies. This symbiotic relationship unveils a profound understanding that bridges the gap between the cosmic and the healing realms, inviting us to explore the intricate threads that weave the universe and human health into a harmonious tapestry.

Astrology attributes specific qualities and attributes to planets, signs, and houses. These cosmic archetypes extend beyond celestial interpretation, finding their counterpart in the homeopathic materia medica. Remedies' archetypal qualities, much like the symbolic associations of heavenly bodies, are believed to resonate with the multifaceted aspects of the human experience physical, emotional, and spiritual.

The dynamic interplay between astrological archetypes and homeopathic remedies provides a nuanced framework for understanding health and well-being. The Sun's representation of vitality and consciousness, for example, aligns with treatments that seek to restore energy and vibrancy within the body.

This resonance goes beyond the surface, delving into the inherent life force that connects the cosmos to individual existence. As we explore the harmonious interplay between celestial archetypes and homeopathic remedies, a deeper understanding of the intricate connections that weave the fabric of health and wholeness emerges.

The alignment of symbolism between planets and remedies offers a unique layer of resonance that supports the healing journey. For instance, the Moon's association with emotions corresponds with homeopathic remedies that address emotional imbalances. A treatment resonating with lunar attributes might be chosen to provide solace during times of heightened emotional sensitivity. This interweaving of cosmic symbolism with healing intentions acknowledges the intricate dance between the emotional and physical aspects of health.

The synergy between planetary archetypes and homeopathic remedies invites a holistic approach to wellness. This approach recognizes that health is not merely the absence of symptoms but the harmonious alignment of the body, mind, and spirit. By selecting remedies that resonate with specific planetary energies, practitioners tap into a deep wellspring of wisdom that echoes across the cosmos, guiding the healing journey toward balance and vitality.

Just as the positions of planets at the moment of birth shape one's astrological blueprint, the resonance between planetary symbolism and remedies underscores the belief in a unique healing blueprint for each individual. This recognition that each person's journey towards well-being is profoundly personal and interconnected with the cosmic order adds a profound dimension to the art of healing.

The alignment between planetary archetypes and homeopathic remedies empowers practitioners and patients. Practitioners gain a richer toolkit to address imbalances and promote healing, drawing upon the wisdom of both the cosmos and the healing arts. Patients, in turn, receive a more comprehensive approach that acknowledges their holistic nature and the interplay between their internal and external worlds.

Conclusion: Celestial Threads of Well-Being:

As we traverse the celestial symphony that harmonizes planetary influences and homeopathic healing, we glimpse the intricate threads that connect the universe's vast expanse with the intimate realm of individual health. The resonance between planetary archetypes and remedies underscores the ancient belief that humanity is intricately woven into the cosmic fabric, a microcosm of the macrocosm. Through this exploration, we honor the dance between the celestial and the human, acknowledging the profound connection that guides us on the journey toward well-being and wholeness.

Healing through Symbolic Correspondences:

The alignment of symbolism between planets and remedies adds a unique resonance layer to support the healing journey. For example, the Moon's association with emotions corresponds with homeopathic remedies targeting emotional imbalances. A treatment resonating with lunar attributes might be chosen to offer solace during times of heightened emotional sensitivity.

This connection between celestial bodies and remedies isn't just symbolic; it's believed to operate on a vibrational level. Just as planets' positions at birth are thought to influence traits, remedies' energetic vibrations align with specific aspects of health. This holistic approach extends healing beyond physical symptoms to emotional and mental well-being.

Planetary Influences on Health Patterns:

Astrology suggests planetary positions at birth influence health tendencies. Homeopathy parallels this by linking specific remedies to planets governing bodily systems. For instance, therapies related to Mars might target conditions involving inflammation, reflecting the planet's fiery nature and its influence on health.

Celestial bodies become metaphors for energetic forces within the body. Mars, associated with heat and action, mirrors the body's response to inflammation. Remedies attributed to Mars hold vibrational imprints resonating with the body's ability to restore balance in inflammation.

The blend of celestial symbolism and healing qualities creates a potent alchemical mixture. Remedies are selected not just for physical attributes but for the deeper resonance within the cosmic order. This alchemy offers a multidimensional healing experience, addressing layers of an individual's constitution and well-being.

This blending aligns with resonance – where similar vibrations interact and influence each other. Remedies' vibrational essences communicate with the body's intelligence, supporting it in recognizing and rectifying imbalances. The result is a holistic approach stimulating the body's healing mechanisms.

Astrology and homeopathy converge in personalized healing. An astrological birth chart provides insight into an individual's cosmic blueprint, while homeopathy tailors remedies to the constitution, symptoms, and imbalances. This aligns with the wisdom that each person embodies a microcosm of the universe.

This perspective recognizes individuals as dynamic beings influenced by various factors. Homeopathy's remedy selection resonates with astrology's belief in a distinctive cosmic imprint shaping each person's journey.

Holistic Insights and Comprehensive Healing:

The symbiosis of symbols offers holistic insights into interconnected existence. Human beings are interconnected with the cosmos, enriching healing by considering physical manifestations and emotional, mental, and spiritual aspects.

Approaching healing holistically acknowledges that health is more than the absence of disease; it's balance and alignment with universal energies. Just as celestial bodies maintain harmonious orbits, individuals seek equilibrium in physical, emotional, and energetic forces.

Astrological symbolism and homeopathic remedies form a fusion of ancient wisdom. This synthesis encourages practitioners to explore beyond conventions, incorporating cosmic insights and vibrational healing. This fusion deepens our understanding of the interplay between universal energies and the human journey.

Practitioners bridge the cosmic and individual, weaving narratives of celestial bodies and health intricacies. This enriches healing, offering a perspective honoring connections between aspects of existence.

The Healing Dance:

Embracing symbiosis, we transcend time and space, recognizing energies within as a dance. As celestial bodies move in intricate patterns, so do energies within us. This allows us to step into the rhythm of this cosmic dance, tapping into the wisdom of the universe and healing arts.

This dance requires attunement to subtle vibrations echoing through the universe, manifesting in planetary archetypes and remedy signatures. Practitioners invite patients into this dance, participants in the symphony of existence. Through this dance, we co-create wellness, resonance, and vibrant health.

Now, let's go deeper into the various astrological signs.

Aries Overview:

Aries individuals, born between March 21 and April 19, belong to the Mars domain, associated with war and desire. Represented by the Ram, Aries is a Fire sign, embodying dynamic energy and boundless enthusiasm. As a Cardinal sign, they are natural leaders and pioneers.

Attributes:

Aries individuals are fearless, determined, and confident. They thrive on challenges and often take the lead in various situations. Their assertiveness can sometimes verge on aggression. They have a spontaneous streak that might lead to risky decisions, but their resilience helps them overcome obstacles.

Mythological References:

Aries is linked to the Golden Ram of Greek mythology, sent by Zeus to save Phrixus and Helle from sacrifice. This ram later became the Aries constellation.

Archetypal References:

Aries embodies the archetype of the Warrior or Hero. They are champions, early adopters, and courageous souls who venture into the unknown. Their purpose-driven attitude and fighting spirit align with mythological warriors and heroes.

Notable Traits:

Under Mars' influence, Aries exudes energy, bravery, and vitality. They initiate actions, often catalyzing projects or defending causes they believe in. Their competitive nature makes them excel in challenging environments.

Additional Information:

As the first zodiac sign, Aries symbolizes beginnings and initiations. They possess an independent spirit, preferring to carve their paths rather than follow established ones.

Taurus Overview:

Taurus individuals, born between April 20 and May 20, are ruled by Venus, linked to affection and aesthetics. With the Bull as their symbol, Taurus is an Earth sign, representing reliability, patience, and a taste for luxury. Their Fixed modality signifies their steadfast yet steady nature.

Attributes:

Taureans are known for loyalty, practicality, and determination. They are builders of the zodiac, laying foundations and seeing tasks through. While dependable, they can be stubborn and resistant to changes that disrupt their comfort.

Mythological References:

The story of Zeus and Europa is tied to Taurus. Zeus transformed into a majestic bull to carry Europa away, later revealing his divine form.

Archetypal References:

Taurus aligns with the Builder or Earth Mother archetype. They symbolize stability, nurturing, and the creation of lasting structures, both physical and metaphorical.

Notable Traits:

Influenced by Venus, Taureans have an innate appreciation for art, beauty, and material comforts. Their senses are heightened, leading them to savor tactile and sensory experiences deeply.

Taurus, associated with material comforts, approaches life pragmatically, ensuring that hard work yields tangible rewards. Their connection to Earth grounds them and fosters a strong affinity for nature.

Gemini Overview:

Gemini, born between May 21 and June 20, is guided by Mercury, linked to communication and cognition. Represented by the Twins, this Air sign signifies adaptability, curiosity, and duality. Their Mutable nature highlights their versatility and spontaneous spirit.

Attributes:

Geminis are optimistic, intellectual, and perpetually curious. Their minds are in constant motion, making them avid gatherers and sharers of information. This dual sign can display unpredictable shifts in mood or opinion.

Mythological References:

Gemini traces back to the Greek twins Castor and Pollux, where one was mortal and the other divine. After Castor's death, Pollux's grief united them in the heavens.

Archetypal References:

Gemini embodies the Messenger or Communicator archetype. Their ability to convey ideas, bridge gaps, and gather information aligns them with mythological messengers or emissaries.

Notable Traits:

With Mercury's influence, Geminis possesses exceptional linguistic skills. They excel in communication-centric professions like journalism or public relations and are brilliant conversationalists.

Gemini's duality enables them to view situations from multiple angles. Their thirst for new experiences and ideas positions them as perpetual students of life.

Cancer Overview:

Cancer individuals, born between June 21 and July 22, are ruled by the Moon, symbolizing emotions and intuition. Represented by the Crab, Cancer is a Water sign, embodying sensitivity, nurturing, and deep emotional connections. Their Cardinal nature marks their initiative and leadership in emotional matters.

Attributes:

Cancerians are known for their vital emotional intelligence, loyalty, and caring nature. They excel in creating a secure and loving environment for themselves and those around them. Occasionally, their emotions can lead to mood swings and a tendency to hold onto the past.

Mythological References:

Cancer is linked to the tale of Hercules battling the Hydra, where the crab emerged as a loyal ally. This story exemplifies Cancer's protective and supportive qualities.

Archetypal References:

Cancer embodies the Caregiver or Nurturer archetype. They are natural protectors, often assuming roles that involve nurturing and fostering growth.

Notable Traits:

Guided by the Moon, Cancerians possess an innate understanding of emotions. Their ability to empathize and provide emotional support strengthens them in relationships.

Cancerians often have strong ties to family and home. They create a sense of security in their surroundings and find comfort in traditions and sentimental values.

Leo Overview:

Leos, born between July 23 and August 22, is ruled by the Sun, symbolizing self-expression and vitality. Represented by the Lion, Leo is a Fire sign, embodying creativity, leadership, and a vibrant personality. Their Fixed nature signifies determination and steadfastness.

Attributes:

Leos are celebrated for their confidence, charisma, and generosity. They have a natural flair for the dramatic and enjoy being at the center of attention. Occasionally, their desire for recognition can lead to arrogance or a need for constant validation.

Mythological References:

Leo is often associated with the Nemean Lion, a beast Hercules conquered as part of his labors. This story mirrors Leo's regal and courageous qualities.

Archetypal References:

Leo embodies the Ruler or Performer archetype. They have an innate ability to lead and inspire others, often shining brightly in roles that demand attention.

Notable Traits:

Guided by the Sun, Leos radiates energy and enthusiasm. Their creative spirit, combined with their leadership skills, often leads them to the forefront of their endeavors.

Leos has a natural affinity for creativity and the arts. They find joy in self-expression and often leave a lasting impact through their artistic contributions.

Virgo Overview:

Virgos, born between August 23 and September 22, is ruled by Mercury, the planet of communication and intellect. Represented by the Virgin, Virgo is an Earth sign, embodying practicality, analytical thinking, and attention to detail. Their Mutable nature signifies adaptability and resourcefulness.

Attributes:

Virgos are known for their precision, practicality, and strong analytical skills. They have an uncanny ability to notice details that others might overlook. Occasionally, their pursuit of perfection can lead to criticism, both of themselves and others.

Mythological References:

The goddess Astraea, often associated with Virgo, symbolizes justice and innocence. The story of her departure from Earth reflects Virgo's pursuit of purity and order.

Archetypal References:

Virgo embodies the Analyst or Healer archetype. Their meticulous nature and keen sense of observation align with problem-solving and nurturing roles.

Notable Traits:

Under Mercury's influence, Virgos possesses exceptional organizational skills and mental acuity. They excel in tasks that require precision and systematic thinking.

Virgos often find fulfillment in serving and helping others. Their practical approach to life, combined with their empathy, makes them reliable and compassionate friends.

Libra Overview:

Libras, born between September 23 and October 22, is ruled by Venus, symbolizing love and harmony. Represented by the Scales, Libra is an Air sign, embodying diplomacy, partnership, and a keen sense of justice. Their Cardinal nature marks their initiative in seeking balance and harmony.

Attributes:

Libras are celebrated for their charm, diplomacy, and ability to foster harmony in relationships. They have a natural talent for mediating conflicts and seeking common ground. Occasionally, their desire for balance can lead to indecision or a tendency to avoid confrontation.

Mythological References:

Libra is often linked to the goddess Themis, representing divine law and order. The symbol of the Scales reflects Libra's pursuit of equilibrium and justice.

Archetypal References:

Libra embodies the Diplomat or Peacemaker archetype. Their ability to bridge gaps and facilitate cooperation aligns them with negotiation and harmony roles.

Notable Traits:

Guided by Venus, Libras possess a refined aesthetic sense and a penchant for cultivating beauty in their surroundings. Their social skills make them adept at building and maintaining connections.

The quest for fairness and harmony drives Libras. They often find joy in creative pursuits and seek balance in their lives.

Scorpio Overview:

Scorpio individuals, born between October 23 and November 21, are ruled by Pluto, symbolizing transformation and depth. Represented by the Scorpion, Scorpio is a Water sign, signifying profound emotions, passion, and determination. Being a Fixed sign, they exhibit steadfastness, determination, and, at times, a hint of secrecy.

Attributes:

Scorpios are celebrated for their intense nature, marked by passion and their ability to penetrate the mysteries of the universe. Their loyalty is unwavering, and when provoked, they can become formidable adversaries. Their love can sometimes manifest as possessiveness or jealousy.

Mythological References:

Scorpio's origins are linked to the story of Orion, the hunter. Boasting that he could eliminate all Earth's animals, he faced a scorpion dispatched to defeat him. The ensuing battle immortalized both in the stars.

Archetypal References:

The Detective or Transformer archetype aligns with Scorpio. They seek truth, immersing themselves in mysteries and delighting in change and renewal.

Notable Traits:

Influenced by Pluto, Scorpios possess a deep understanding of life's enigmas. Their magnetic charm and knack for seeing through facades make them intriguing and somewhat intimidating.

Scorpios exhibit an uncanny knack for rebirth and regeneration. Their journey often leads them through emotional depths, resulting in profound personal transformations.

Sagittarius Overview:

Sagittarians, born between November 22 and December 21, are governed by Jupiter, the planet of expansion and knowledge. Represented by the Archer or Centaur, Sagittarius is a Fire sign, exuding enthusiasm, adventure, and an insatiable thirst for knowledge. Their Mutable nature highlights adaptability and curiosity.

Attributes:

Sagittarians are renowned for their optimism, love of travel, and philosophical outlook. They're natural explorers both intellectually and geographically. Their free spirit can sometimes come across as restlessness or tactlessness.

Mythological References:

The centaur Chiron, a knowledgeable healer and teacher, often symbolizes Sagittarius. His wisdom and adventurous spirit capture the essence of the Sagittarian archetype.

Archetypal References:

Sagittarius embodies the Explorer or Philosopher archetype. Their boundless quest for truth and knowledge resonates with the sages and wanderers of countless myths.

Notable Traits:

Guided by Jupiter, Sagittarians possess a restless spirit, always seeking to broaden their horizons. Their love for adventure frequently leads them to explore new terrains, both physical and intellectual.

Sagittarians are often drawn to fields that allow them to expand their knowledge base and share their wisdom, whether through teaching, writing, or other forms of communication.

Capricorn Overview:

Capricorns, born between December 22 and January 19, are ruled by Saturn, the planet of discipline and structure. Symbolized by the Mountain Goat, Capricorn is an Earth sign, epitomizing practicality, ambition, and resilience. As a Cardinal sign, they exhibit leadership and a systematic approach to life.

Attributes:

Capricorns are recognized for their discipline, patience, and strategic thinking. They possess a long-term vision and work tirelessly to achieve their objectives. At times, their focus on achievement may cause them to seem distant or overly severe.

Mythological References:

Capricorn is often associated with the deity Pan, the god of the wild, shepherds, and rustic music. His resilience and connection to nature mirror the enduring nature of Capricorns.

Archetypal References:

Capricorn aligns with the Builder or Organizer archetype. Their penchant for structure, discipline, and long-term planning resonates with the architects and master planners of various legends.

Notable Traits:

Under Saturn's influence, Capricorns exhibit a mature outlook on life. Their determination, combined with their pragmatic approach, often propels them to positions of leadership and authority.

Capricorns hold tradition in high regard and typically deeply respect the past. Their disciplined nature, coupled with their ambition, fuels their relentless pursuit of goals.

Aquarius Overview:

Aquarians, born between January 20 and February 18, are ruled by Uranus, the planet of innovation and rebellion. Represented by the Water Bearer, Aquarius is an Air sign, symbolizing intellect, uniqueness, and humanitarian ideals. Their Fixed nature underscores their determination and persistence.

Attributes:

Aquarians are known for their intellectual prowess, originality, and unwavering commitment to social causes. They thrive on breaking barriers and challenging norms. Occasionally, their detachment from emotions can lead to perceived aloofness.

Mythological References:

Aquarius is often linked to Ganymede, a handsome mortal carried to Mount Olympus by an eagle to serve as Zeus's cupbearer. This story mirrors the Water Bearer's role of bringing knowledge and enlightenment.

Archetypal References:

Aquarius embodies the Visionary or Humanitarian archetype. They're catalysts for change, ushering in new ideas and pushing boundaries for the betterment of society.

Notable Traits:

Under Uranus' influence, Aquarians possess an unmatched ability to think outside the box. Their innovative thinking and concern for humanity often lead them to become advocates for social progress.

Aquarians often feel a sense of duty towards humanity. Pursuing a better world drives them, and they often find themselves at the forefront of social movements.

Pisces Overview:

Pisceans, born between February 19 and March 20, is ruled by Neptune, the planet of dreams and spirituality. Symbolized by the Fish, Pisces is a Water sign, signifying intuition, empathy, and a deep connection to the mystical. Their Mutable nature marks their adaptability and artistic inclination.

Attributes:

Pisceans are celebrated for their empathetic nature, artistic talents, and profound emotional depth. They have an innate ability to understand others' feelings but sometimes struggle with setting boundaries, leading to emotional vulnerability.

Mythological References:

Pisces ties back to the story of Aphrodite and Eros, who transformed into fish to escape the monster Typhon. This tale exemplifies Pisces' themes of escape, spirituality, and the fluidity of emotions.

Archetypal References:

Pisces embodies the Artist or Mystic archetype. Their connection to the ethereal realms, combined with their creative expression, aligns with the essence of artistic and spiritual guides.

Notable Traits:

Guided by Neptune, Pisceans possess a heightened sense of intuition and imagination. Their artistic talents often manifest in various forms, from visual arts to music.

Pisceans are deeply attuned to the unseen realms. Their spiritual inclinations and sensitivity make them compassionate souls who often find solace in creative pursuits.

What follows is a very detailed list of challenging characteristics associated with each planet. After which follows a list of homeopathic remedies which are best suited to deal with these peculiarities

Disclaimer: This is not to be taken as medical advice. This is for purely entertainment purposes only. If you're experiencing any of these difficulties, challenges, or symptoms, please consult a licensed, qualified healthcare practitioner.

When reviewing persons, natal, and astrology charts, if any of these planets are presented in overwhelming, challenging aspects, it might be interesting to look at the various homeopathic remedies that may be helpful along with many other factors.

Challenging characteristics of the Sun

Egotistical, Dominant, Overexerted, Overconfident, Sensitive, Validation-seeking, Self-centered, Impatient, Competitive, Inflexible, Arrogant, Unyielding, Brash, Spotlight-hungry, Dogmatic, Uncompromising, Boastful, Oblivious, Rigid, Inattentive, Pretentious, Unempathetic, Dictatorial, Overbearing, Grandiose, Intolerant, Impulsive, Unreceptive, Vainglorious, Exaggerative.

Homeopathic Remedies:

• Aconite (Aconitum napellus): Often used for sudden and intense symptoms triggered by cold wind or shock. Beneficial for impatience, intolerance, or impulsiveness.

• Argentum nitricum: Commonly recommended for anxiety with apprehension and hurriedness. Helpful for impulsiveness, overexertion, or inattentiveness.

• Lycopodium (Lycopodium clavatum): A remedy for lack of confidence, potentially appearing overconfident. Suitable for traits like egotism, boasting, or pretentiousness.

• Nux vomica: For ambitious individuals becoming impatient or angered when things don't go their way. Can temper dominance, competitiveness, and rigidity.

• Staphysagria: Addresses bottling up emotions, appearing pleasant but holding pent-up feelings. Beneficial for sensitivity to criticism or validation-seeking.

• Platinum metallic: For viewing oneself as superior or exhibiting arrogance.

• Aurum metallicum: Often used for deep feelings of worthlessness or feeling unforgivable. Beneficial for being overly self-centered or dictatorial.

• Pulsatilla (Pulsatilla pratensis): For soft-hearted individuals seeking attention and validation. It can temper spotlight-hungry or validation-seeking tendencies.

• Sulphur: For intellectual individuals absorbed in ideas, theories, or dogma. Suitable for traits like rigidity, inflexibility, or obliviousness.

• Baryta carbonica: Helpful for lack of confidence and shyness, occasionally overcompensating with arrogance or boasting.

Challenging characteristics of the Moon:

Moodiness, Emotional Fluctuation, Erratic Behavior, Heightened Emotional Reactions, Amplified Sensitivity, Overreaction, Difficulty with Criticisms, Difficulty Letting Go of the Past, Holding On to People, Overly Nostalgic, Clingy, Indecisiveness, Difficult Rational Decision-making, Overly Intuitive, Overly Attached, Need for Emotional Security, Possessiveness, Dependence on People, Vulnerability, Easily Hurt, Affected by External Influences, Overly Emotionally Protective, Escapist, Escapism, Difficulty Managing, Intense Feelings, Overly Sympathetic, Psychic, Resist Change, Clings to Familiar, Poor Decision Making.

Homeopathic Remedies:

• Pulsatilla: For emotional fluctuations and heightened reactions. It helps those who are overly sensitive and tend to overreact emotionally.

• Natrum Muriaticum: Addresses difficulty letting go of the past and holding onto people. Beneficial for sensitivity and need for security.

• Lycopodium: For indecisiveness and emotional attachment. Helps with vulnerability and sensitivity to criticism.

• Ignatia: Useful for intense feelings and emotional fluctuations. It can help with resistance to change and attachment to the familiar.

• Sepia: Suits those struggling with poor decision-making and emotions. Addresses escapism and emotional vulnerability.

• Arsenicum Album: For intense feelings and need for emotional security. Beneficial for attachment and escapist tendencies.

• Phosphorus: For sensitivity to external influences and poor decision-making. Helps with emotional reactions and security needs.

• Calcarea Carbonica: Addresses emotional attachment and dependence. Beneficial for vulnerability and need for stability.

• Staphysagria: For difficulty letting go and emotional attachment. Helps with sensitivity and security needs.

• Lachesis: Useful for intense feelings and resistance to change. Addresses vulnerability and emotional needs.

Challenging Characteristics of Mercury:

Communication issues, Nervousness, Restlessness, Overthinking, Worry, Inconsistency, Shyness, Difficulty concentrating, Impatience, being overwhelmed by details, Tendency to jump to conclusions, Nervous habits, Quick decision-making, Lack of follow-through, Anxiousness, Mental agitation, Difficulty listening actively, Fear of making mistakes.

Homeopathic Remedies for Mercury Characteristics:

• Argentum Nitricum: May struggle with nervousness and communication issues. Exhibits restlessness and overthinking. Addresses the tendency to jump to conclusions and mental agitation.

• Gelsemium: Suits those with communication issues and nervousness. Overwhelmed by details and exhibits shyness. Addresses difficulty concentrating and alleviates anxiousness.

• Natrum Muriaticum: Experiences restlessness and worry. He struggles with overthinking and shyness. Addresses the tendency to jump to conclusions and alleviates mental agitation.

• Lycopodium: Exhibits difficulty concentrating and impatience. Experiences restlessness and overthinking. Addresses quick decision-making and lack of follow-through.

• Pulsatilla: Struggles with communication issues and shyness. Experiences inconsistency and worry. Addresses difficulty listening actively and alleviates the fear of making mistakes.

• Arsenicum Album: Experiences nervousness and mental agitation. Difficulty concentrating and being overwhelmed by details. Addresses impatience and alleviates anxiousness.

• Nux Vomica: Exhibits restlessness and impatience. She struggles with communication issues and overthinking. Addresses quick decision-making and alleviates mental agitation.

• Silicea: Struggles with difficulty concentrating and shyness. Overwhelmed by details and worry. Addresses the tendency to jump to conclusions and alleviates anxiousness.

Challenging Characteristics of Venus:

Indecisiveness, Overindulgence, Superficiality, Dependency on others for validation, Insecurity in relationships, Difficulty asserting oneself, Fear of rejection, Jealousy, Tendency to avoid confrontation, Overspending, Self-doubt, Excessive people-pleasing, Vanity, Unrealistic romantic ideals, Over-emphasis on physical appearance.

Homeopathic Remedies for Venus Characteristics:

• Pulsatilla: Struggles with indecisiveness and dependency on others for validation. Exhibits insecurity in relationships and avoids confrontation. Addresses people-pleasing tendencies and alleviates self-doubt.

• Natrum Muriaticum: Difficulty asserting oneself and struggles with insecurity in relationships. Exhibits fear of rejection and superficiality. Addresses the tendency to avoid confrontation and alleviates self-doubt.

• Lycopodium: Experiences overindulgence and dependency on others for validation. Exhibits insecurity in relationships and indecisiveness. It addresses vanity and unrealistic romantic ideals.

• Calcarea Carbonica: Struggles with indecisiveness and overindulgence. Exhibits insecurity in relationships and dependency on others for validation. Addresses self-doubt and tendency to avoid confrontation.

• Ignatia: Difficulty asserting oneself and exhibits insecurity in relationships. Struggles with fear of rejection and self-doubt. Addresses excessive people-pleasing tendencies.

• Arsenicum Album: Difficulty asserting oneself and insecurity in relationships. Exhibits superficiality and indecisiveness. Addresses fear of rejection and alleviates self-doubt.

• Lachesis: Struggles with jealousy and dependency on others for validation. Exhibits insecurity in relationships and indecisiveness. Addresses the tendency to avoid confrontation and alleviates self-doubt.

• Silicea: Difficulty asserting oneself and insecurity in relationships. Exhibits overindulgence and indecisiveness. Addresses fear of rejection and unrealistic romantic ideals.

Challenging Characteristics of Jupiter:

Excessive optimism, Overindulgence, Impulsiveness, Overconfidence, Tendency to take on too much, Disregard for details, Restlessness, Laziness, Overextending oneself, Extravagance,

Self-righteousness, Arrogance, Inflated ego, Lack of practicality, Overcommitting, Overpromising.

Homeopathic Remedies for Jupiter Characteristics:

• Lycopodium: Struggles with overindulgence and excessive optimism. Exhibits overconfidence and a tendency to take on too much. Addresses lack of practicality and alleviates laziness.

• Nux Vomica: Suits those with impulsiveness and may struggle with overindulgence. Exhibits overconfidence and disregard for details. It helps address restlessness and the tendency to overextend.

• Calcarea Carbonica: Experiences laziness and lack of practicality. Struggles with overindulgence and restlessness. Addresses taking on too much and alleviates self-righteousness.

• Ignatia: Tends to take on too much and may exhibit excessive optimism. Experiences impulsiveness and restlessness. Addresses lack of practicality and alleviates overcommitting tendencies.

• Arsenicum Album: Struggles with overconfidence and overindulgence. Exhibits laziness and disregard for details. Addresses extravagance and tendency to overpromise.

• Pulsatilla: Tends to take on too much and may struggle with overindulgence. Experiences laziness and overconfidence. It helps address a lack of practicality and alleviates self-righteousness.

• Chamomilla: Experiences impulsiveness and restlessness. He struggles with overindulgence and a tendency to take on too much. Addresses arrogance and alleviates lack of practicality.

• Natrum Muriaticum: Exhibits overconfidence and may struggle with overindulgence. Experiences laziness and restlessness. It helps address taking on too much and alleviates self-righteousness.

Challenging Characteristics of Saturn:

Fear of failure, Pessimism, Self-doubt, Insecurity, Overwhelming responsibility, Rigidity, Fear of change, Perfectionism, Isolation, Difficulty expressing emotions, Self-criticism, Impatience,

Stubbornness, Overwork, Tendency to hold onto grudges, Harsh self-discipline.

Homeopathic Remedies for Saturn Characteristics:

• Aurum: Struggles with self-doubt and fear of failure. Experiences overwhelming responsibility and perfectionism. Addresses the tendency to isolate and alleviates fear of change.

• Natrum Muriaticum: Exhibits insecurity and self-doubt. Struggles with fear of failure and rigidity. It helps address difficulty expressing emotions and alleviates pessimism.

• Arsenicum Album: Experiences self-doubt and insecurity. Struggles with perfectionism and fear of change. Addresses fear of failure and tendency to hold onto grudges.

• Lycopodium: Has a fear of failure and may exhibit self-doubt. Experiences rigidity and overwhelming responsibility. It helps address self-criticism and alleviates impatience.

• Nux Vomica: Struggles with pessimism and insecurity. Experiences overwork and rigidity. Addresses the tendency to hold onto grudges and alleviates impatience.

• Causticum: Exhibits difficulty expressing emotions and insecurity. Struggles with rigidity and fear of change. Addresses fear of failure and alleviates harsh self-discipline.

• Sepia: Experiences self-doubt and insecurity. Struggles with isolation and perfectionism. It helps address difficulty expressing emotions and alleviates pessimism.

• Staphysagria: Struggles with insecurity and fear of failure. Experiences self-doubt and perfectionism. Addresses stubbornness and alleviates fear of change.

Challenging Characteristics of Uranus:

Rebellion for the sake of rebellion, Restlessness, Impatience with routine, Disregard for tradition, Eccentric behavior, Abrupt changes, over-idealism, Impulsiveness, Tendency to shock or provoke, Difficulty with commitment, Disruptive tendencies, Unpredictability, Disconnection from emotions, Resistance to authority.

Homeopathic Remedies for Challenging Uranus Characteristics:

Pulsatilla: Pulsatilla individuals may exhibit restlessness and impulsiveness. They can struggle with over-idealism and a tendency to provoke. This remedy can address their difficulty with commitment and alleviate their disconnect from emotions.

Aconitum: Aconitum suits those who have impulsiveness and may exhibit restlessness. They can struggle with abrupt changes and over-idealism. This remedy can help address their tendency to shock and alleviate their resistance to authority.

Arsenicum Album: Arsenicum Album individuals may experience restlessness and impatience with routine. They can struggle with eccentric behavior and disruptive tendencies. This remedy can address their unpredictability and alleviate they are over idealism.

Ignatia: Ignatia suits those with difficulty with commitment and may exhibit restlessness. They can struggle with impulsive behavior and over-idealism. This remedy can help address their disconnection from emotions and alleviate their tendency to provoke.

Nux Vomica: Nux Vomica individuals may exhibit impatience with routine and restlessness. They can struggle with abrupt changes and impulsiveness. This remedy can address their resistance to authority and alleviate their over-idealism.

Natrum Muriaticum: Natrum Muriaticum suits those who tend to provoke and may experience restlessness. They can struggle with eccentric behavior and impulsiveness. This remedy can help address their disconnect from emotions and alleviate their resistance to authority.

Lachesis: Lachesis individuals may experience impatience with routine and restlessness. They can struggle with abrupt changes and eccentric behavior. This remedy can address their tendency to shock or provoke and alleviate their over-idealism.

Sulphur: Sulphur suits those who have impulsiveness and may struggle with restlessness. They can exhibit disruptive tendencies and eccentric behavior. This remedy can help address their resistance to authority and alleviate their over-idealism.

Challenging Characteristics of Neptune:

Illusions, Delusions, Escapism, Confusion, Deception, Disorganization, Vulnerability to addiction, Unrealistic ideals, Over-sensitivity, Lack of boundaries, Self-sacrifice, Tendency to avoid confrontation, Idealizing others, Clouded perception, Emotional turmoil, Lack of focus.

Homeopathic Remedies for Challenging, Neptune Characteristics:

Natrum Muriaticum: Muriaticum individuals may struggle with over-sensitivity and lack of boundaries. They can experience confusion and vulnerability to addiction. This remedy can address their tendency to avoid confrontation and alleviate their idealizing preferences.

Pulsatilla: Pulsatilla suits those who have over-sensitivity and may struggle with confusion. They can exhibit unrealistic ideals and a lack of boundaries. This remedy can help address their tendency to avoid confrontation and alleviate their vulnerability to addiction.

Arsenicum Album: Arsenicum Album individuals may experience confusion and unrealistic ideals. They can struggle with over-sensitivity and self-sacrifice. This remedy can address their emotional turmoil and alleviate their lack of boundaries.

Sepia: Sepia suits those who lack boundaries and may struggle with confusion. They can experience emotional turmoil and over-sensitivity. This remedy can help address their vulnerability to addiction and alleviate their tendency to idealize others.

Lachesis: Lachesis individuals may experience unrealistic ideals and a lack of boundaries. They can struggle with over-sensitivity and self-sacrifice. This remedy can address their clouded perception and alleviate their tendency to avoid confrontation.

Stramonium: Stramonium suits those who have confusion and may struggle with a lack of boundaries. They can experience emotional turmoil and vulnerability to addiction. This remedy can help address their tendency to idealize others and alleviate their delusions.

Phosphoric Acid: Phosphoric Acid individuals may experience disorganization and confusion. They can struggle with a lack of focus and vulnerability to addiction. This remedy can address their tendency to escape and alleviate their clouded perception.

Cannabis Indica: Cannabis Indica suits those who are confused and may struggle with a lack of boundaries. They can experience disorganization and vulnerability to addiction. This remedy can help address their escapist tendencies and alleviate their unrealistic ideals.

Challenging Characteristics of Pluto:

Obsessions, Power struggles, Control issues, Fear of vulnerability, Intense emotions, Resentment, Transformational upheaval, Manipulation, Destructive behavior, Stubbornness, Fear of change, Difficulty letting go, Fixations, Need for secrecy, Deep-seated fears.

Homeopathic Remedies for Challenging Pluto Characteristics:

Lachesis: Lachesis individuals may struggle with power struggles and control issues. They can exhibit fear of vulnerability and intense emotions. This remedy can address their tendency for manipulation and alleviate their anxiety about change.

Natrum Muriaticum: Natrum Muriaticum suits those who fear vulnerability and may struggle with fixations. They can experience resentment and intense emotions. This remedy can help address their fear of change and alleviate their control issues.

Sepia: Sepia suits those who have difficulty letting go and may struggle with fixations. They can experience intense emotions and power struggles. This remedy can address their fear of vulnerability and alleviate their stubbornness.

Thuja Occidentalis: Thuja Occidentalis individuals may experience fear of vulnerability and change. They can struggle with power struggles and control issues. This remedy can help address their need for secrecy and alleviate their fixations.

Staphysagria: Staphysagria suits those with power struggles and may struggle with fear of vulnerability. They can experience intense emotions and fear of change. This remedy can address their tendency for manipulation and alleviate their destructive behavior.

Arsenicum Album: Arsenicum Album individuals may experience fear of vulnerability and control issues. They can struggle with intense emotions and power struggles. This remedy can help address their need for secrecy and alleviate their fixations.

Carcinosinum: Carcinosinum suits those who have a fear of vulnerability and fear of change. They can struggle with obsessions and control issues. This remedy can address their deep-seated fears and alleviate their manipulative tendencies.

Ignatia: Ignatia individuals may experience intense emotions and difficulty letting go. They can struggle with fear of vulnerability and power struggles. This remedy can help address their resentment and alleviate their fixations.

Chiron:

Challenging Characteristics: Wounds, Insecurity, Deep emotional pain, Feelings of inadequacy, Unhealed trauma, Vulnerabilities.

Homeopathic Remedies: As Chiron represents wounds and healing, there isn't a direct correlation to homeopathic remedies. Healing work and therapies would be more relevant.

Ceres:

Challenging Characteristics: Dependency, Over-nurturing, Perceived loss of control, Emotional manipulation, Difficulty finding balance.

Homeopathic Remedies: Ceres are associated with nurturing and sustenance, so remedies that support emotional balance, such as Natrum Muriaticum or Pulsatilla, might be relevant.

Juno:

Challenging Characteristics: Codependency, Unhealthy attachments, Difficulty asserting oneself in relationships, Fear of betrayal.

Homeopathic Remedies: Juno's themes are primarily relationship-oriented, so remedies that address communication and emotional balance, like Ignatia or Natrum Muriaticum, could be considered.

Pallas Athena:

Challenging Characteristics: Overthinking, Analysis paralysis, Difficulty finding creative solutions, Lack of strategic thinking.

Homeopathic Remedies: Pallas Athena is associated with wisdom and strategy, so remedies that support mental clarity and focus, such as Lycopodium or Nux Vomica, could be relevant.

Vesta:

Challenging Characteristics: Workaholism, Over-committing to duties, Difficulty maintaining work-life balance, Neglecting personal needs.

Homeopathic Remedies: Vesta's themes are linked to dedication and focus, so remedies that address balance and stress management, like Sepia or Aurum, might be considered.

North Node:

Challenging Characteristics: Resistance to growth, Stagnation, Fear of change, Staying within comfort zones, Avoidance of life lessons.

Homeopathic Remedies: The North Node represents the growth path, so remedies that support adaptability and embracing change, like Arsenicum Album or Lachesis, might be relevant.

Disclaimer: All information regarding homeopathic medicine is to be considered for entertainment purposes only. No medical advice has been given in any way. If you have concerns about your health, please contact a qualified healthcare practitioner of your choice.

Completed List of Challenging Characteristics of each sign and Remedies that might help in these challenging characteristics and symptomology.

Challenging Characteristics of Aries:

Impulsiveness, Impatience, Recklessness, Quick temper, Impulsive decision-making, Self-centeredness, Lack of consideration for others, Competitive nature, Restlessness, Difficulty following through, Aggression, Tendency to jump into action without thinking, Poor listening skills, Stubbornness, Overbearing behavior, Lack of patience, Need for constant stimulation, Tendency to disregard consequences, Need for instant gratification.

Homeopathic Remedies for Aries Characteristics:

Belladonna: Belladonna individuals can be impulsive and have a quick temper. They may exhibit aggression and a lack of patience. This remedy can help address their tendency to jump into action without thinking and the need for instant gratification.

Lycopodium: Lycopodium suits those who are competitive and may be self-centered. They can exhibit impulsive decision-making and overbearing behavior. This remedy can address their impatience and the tendency to disregard consequences.

Nux Vomica: Nux Vomica individuals may have a quick temper and impatience. They may be aggressive and competitive, often lacking patience. This remedy can help address their impulsiveness and the tendency to jump into action without thinking.

Bryonia: Bryonia individuals can be impatient and self-centered. They may exhibit aggression and a competitive nature. This remedy can address their impulsive decision-making and the need for instant gratification.

Chamomilla: Chamomilla suits those with a quick temper and may be self-centered. They can exhibit restlessness and aggression. This remedy can help address their impulsive behavior

Challenging Characteristics of Taurus:

Stubbornness, Resistance to change, Materialistic tendencies, Possessiveness, Attachment to comfort, Inflexibility, Laziness, Resistance to new ideas, Difficulty adapting to change, Overindulgence, Reluctance to take risks, Overemphasis on routine, Over-attachment to possessions, Difficulty letting go, Fear of change, Stagnation, Rigid opinions, Overemphasis on physical comforts, Resistance to change, Difficulty embracing new experiences.

Homeopathic Remedies for Taurus Characteristics:

Calcarea Carbonica: Individuals may exhibit stubbornness and resistance to change. They tend to be materialistic and possessive. This remedy can help address their inflexibility and the overemphasis on physical comforts.

Lycopodium: Suits those who have rigid opinions and may be possessive. They can exhibit materialistic tendencies and resistance to new ideas. This remedy can address their inflexibility and the fear of change.

Nux Vomica: Individuals may struggle with stubbornness and possessiveness. They may resist change and have difficulty adapting. This remedy can help address their rigidity and the overemphasis on routine.

Pulsatilla: Individuals can exhibit attachment to comfort and possessiveness. They may resist new ideas and have difficulty letting go. This remedy can address their reluctance to take risks and fear of change.

Bryonia: Suits those who have inflexibility and materialistic tendencies. They can exhibit possessiveness and attachment to comfort. This remedy can help address their resistance to new ideas and the overemphasis on routine.

Sepia: Individuals may struggle with attachment to comfort and possessiveness. They may resist change and have difficulty letting go. This remedy can help address their inflexibility and the overemphasis on physical comforts.

Ignatia: Individuals may exhibit resistance to change and possessiveness. They can struggle with inflexibility and attachment to comfort. This remedy can address their difficulty adapting and their fear of change.

Silicea: Suits those who have rigid opinions and may be possessive. They can exhibit materialistic tendencies and resistance to new ideas. This remedy can help address their inflexibility and the overemphasis on physical comforts.

Homeopathic Remedies for Taurus Characteristics:

Calcarea Carbonica individuals may exhibit stubbornness and resistance to change. They tend to be materialistic and possessive. This remedy can help address their inflexibility and overemphasis on physical comforts.

Lycopodium: Lycopodium suits those who have rigid opinions and may be possessive. They can exhibit materialistic tendencies and resistance to new ideas. This remedy can address their inflexibility and fear of change.

Nux Vomica: Nux Vomica individuals may struggle with stubbornness and possessiveness. They may resist change and have difficulty adapting. This remedy can help address their rigidity and overemphasis on routine.

Pulsatilla: Pulsatilla individuals can exhibit attachment to comfort and possessiveness. They may resist new ideas and have difficulty letting go. This remedy can address their reluctance to take risks and fear of change.

Bryonia: Bryonia suits those who have inflexibility and materialistic tendencies. They can exhibit possessiveness and attachment to comfort. This remedy can help address their resistance to new ideas and overemphasis on routine.

Sepia: Sepia individuals may struggle with attachment to comfort and possessiveness. They may resist change and have difficulty letting go. This remedy can help address their inflexibility and overemphasis on physical comforts.

Ignatia: Ignatia individuals may exhibit resistance to change and possessiveness. They can struggle with inflexibility and attachment to comfort. This remedy can address their difficulty adapting and fear of change.

Silicea: Silicea suits those who have rigid opinions and may be possessive. They can exhibit materialistic tendencies and resistance to new ideas. This remedy can help address their inflexibility and overemphasis on physical comforts.

Challenging Characteristics of Gemini:

Restlessness, Superficiality, Inconsistency, Gossipy tendencies, Difficulty focusing, Scattered energy, Impatience, Impulsiveness, Lack of follow-through, Nervousness, Shallow relationships, Tendency to jump from topic to topic, Overemphasis on intellectual pursuits, Lack of commitment, short attention span, Difficulty making decisions, Flightiness, Tendency to exaggerate, Overemphasis on socializing, Difficulty sticking to one task, Disregard for practical details.

Homeopathic Remedies for Gemini Characteristics:

Pulsatilla: Pulsatilla individuals may exhibit restlessness and superficiality. They can struggle with inconsistency and scattered energy. This remedy can help address their flightiness and the tendency to jump from topic to topic.

Natrum Muriaticum: Natrum Muriaticum suits those with short attention spans and may be impatient. They can exhibit nervousness and impulsiveness. This remedy can help address their scattered energy and difficulty in focusing.

Lycopodium: Lycopodium individuals may struggle with inconsistency and lack of follow-through. They can be gossipy and have a superficial approach. This remedy can address their flightiness and overemphasis on intellectual pursuits.

Nux Vomica: Nux Vomica suits those who have impatience and impulsiveness. They may struggle with a lack of follow-through and scattered energy. This remedy can help address their short attention span and the tendency to exaggerate.

Silicea: Silicea individuals may exhibit difficulty focusing and inconsistency. They can struggle with restlessness and impatience. This remedy can help address their scattered energy and the tendency to jump from topic to topic.

Gelsemium: Gelsemium suits those with short attention spans and may be impatient. They can exhibit nervousness and lack of follow-through. This remedy can help address their flightiness and difficulty in focusing.

Sepia: Sepia individuals may struggle with inconsistency and lack of follow-through. They can be gossipy and have a superficial approach. This remedy can address their flightiness and overemphasis on socializing.

Chamomilla: Chamomilla suits those who have impatience and impulsiveness. They may struggle with nervousness and scattered energy. This remedy can help address their short attention span and the tendency to exaggerate.

Challenging Characteristics of Cancer:

Overemotional, Moody, Clinginess, Overprotectiveness, Difficulty letting go of the past, Nurturing to the point of self-neglect, Sensitivity to criticism, Fear of rejection, Avoidance of confrontation, Mood swings, Attachment to comfort, Tendency to retreat into the shell, Oversensitivity, Reluctance to show vulnerability, Difficulty setting boundaries, Emotional manipulation, Fear of being hurt, Difficulty expressing emotions, Excessive nostalgia.

Homeopathic Remedies for Cancer Characteristics:

Pulsatilla individuals may exhibit moodiness and clinginess. They can be overly emotional and sensitive to criticism. This remedy can help address their attachment to comfort and the tendency to retreat into the shell.

Natrum Muriaticum suits those who have difficulty letting go of the past and maybe overly sensitive. They can be emotionally withdrawn and fear rejection. This remedy can help address their reluctance to show vulnerability and the tendency to avoid confrontation.

Ignatia individuals may struggle with mood swings and sensitivity to criticism. They can have difficulty setting boundaries and fear of being hurt. This remedy can help address their emotional ups and downs and the tendency to retreat into the shell.

Sepia suits those who have difficulty letting go of the past and may be overprotective. They can struggle with emotional manipulation and avoidance of confrontation. This remedy can help address their sensitivity and reluctance to show vulnerability.

Challenging Characteristics of Leo:

Ego-centeredness, Attention-seeking behavior, Arrogance, need for constant validation, Excessive pride, Self-centeredness, Tendency to dominate, Stubbornness, Resistance to criticism, Overbearing behavior, Dramatic tendencies, Desire for admiration, Reluctance to share the spotlight, Difficulty acknowledging faults, Intolerance of opposition, Overemphasis on appearance, Tendency to be bossy, Impatience with others, Difficulty with humility, Tendency to be demanding.

Homeopathic Remedies for Leo Characteristics:

Lycopodium individuals may exhibit ego-centeredness and attention-seeking behavior. They can be arrogant and need constant validation. This remedy can help address their self-centeredness and the tendency to dominate.

Nux Vomica suits those who tend to be bossy and resist criticism. They can be impatient with others and exhibit dramatic tendencies. This remedy can help address their overbearing behavior and the need for constant validation.

Staphysagria individuals may struggle with excessive pride and self-centeredness. They can have difficulty acknowledging faults and resisting criticism. This remedy can help address their arrogance and the tendency to dominate.

Belladonna suits those with a dramatic tendency and desire for admiration. They can be impatient with others and need constant validation. This remedy can help address their attention-seeking behavior and the tendency to be bossy.

Challenging Characteristics of Virgo:

Perfectionism, Overcritical, Nitpicking, Obsessive-compulsive tendencies, Anxious, Worrisome, Hyper-focused on details, Difficulty seeing the bigger picture, Overanalyzing, Judgmental, Self-critical, Self-doubt, Inflexibility, Rigid expectations, Fear of failure, Excessive orderliness, Prone to health concerns, Hypochondriac tendencies, Overemphasis on cleanliness, Skeptical, Overwhelmed by details, Difficulty delegating, Micromanaging, Tendency to worry about others, Difficulty expressing emotions, Suppressing emotions, Difficulty letting go, Fear of imperfection,

Overemphasis on routine, Need for control, Over-attachment to possessions.

Homeopathic Remedies for Virgo Characteristics:

Natrum Muriaticum: Individuals may exhibit perfectionism and obsessive-compulsive tendencies. They suppress emotions and have a fear of imperfection. This remedy can help address their self-critical nature and the inner tension they experience.

Arsenicum Album Suits those who are pessimistic and fear failure. They may be over-workaholics and suppress emotions. This remedy can help address their anxiety and excessive focus on material success.

Lycopodium Individuals can be overcritical and judgmental. They may have rigid expectations and a fear of criticism. This remedy can help address their self-doubt and tendency to micromanage.

Calcarea Carbonica Suits those who fear change and have difficulty relaxing. They may be over-responsible and suppress emotions. This remedy can help address their anxiety and the tendency to isolate themselves.

Pulsatilla Suits those who have difficulty letting go and fear chaos. They tend to suppress emotions and have a fear of criticism. This remedy can help address their need for emotional expression and the tendency to martyr themselves.

Sepia Individuals may struggle with attachment to comfort and possessiveness. They may resist change and have difficulty letting go. This remedy can help address their inflexibility and the overemphasis on physical comforts.

Ignatia Individuals may exhibit resistance to change and possessiveness. They can struggle with inflexibility and attachment to comfort. This remedy can address their difficulty adapting and their fear of change.

Silicea Suits those who have rigid opinions and may be possessive. They can exhibit materialistic tendencies and resistance to new ideas. This remedy can help address their inflexibility and the overemphasis on physical comforts.

Challenging Characteristics of Libra:

Indecisiveness, People-pleasing tendencies, Difficulty asserting oneself, Avoidance of conflict, Need for harmony at all costs, Superficiality, Overemphasis on appearance, Reluctance to make waves, Tendency to compromise personal needs, Fear of rejection, Overemphasis on partnerships, Difficulty making decisions, Tendency to be passive-aggressive, Reluctance to confront difficult situations, Tendency to be diplomatic to the point of dishonesty, Difficulty setting boundaries, Over-attachment to others' opinions.

Homeopathic Remedies for Libra Characteristics:

Pulsatilla Individuals may struggle with indecisiveness and people-pleasing tendencies. They tend to avoid conflict and have difficulty asserting themselves. This remedy can help address their need for harmony and the tendency to compromise personal needs.

Sepia Suits those who have difficulty asserting themselves and avoiding conflict. They can struggle with over-attachment to others' opinions and the tendency to compromise personal needs. This remedy can help address their reluctance to confront difficult situations.

Lycopodium Individuals may exhibit indecisiveness and superficiality. They can have a fear of rejection and avoid conflict. This remedy can help address their reluctance to make waves and the overemphasis on appearance.

Natrum Muriaticum Suits those who have difficulty asserting themselves and a need for harmony at all costs. They can struggle with superficiality and avoidance of conflict. This remedy can help address their reluctance to confront difficult situations and the tendency to compromise personal needs.

Challenging Characteristics of Scorpio:

Intensity, Obsessiveness, Secretive tendencies, Distrust, Manipulative behavior, Jealousy, Fear of vulnerability, Tendency to hold grudges, Difficulty forgiving, Deep emotional wounds, Need for control, Stubbornness, Tendency to be self-destructive, Vindictiveness, Compulsive behavior, Fear of betrayal, Difficulty letting go, Resentment, Desire for power and control, Emotional volatility.

Homeopathic Remedies for Scorpio Characteristics:

Lachesis Individuals may exhibit intensity and secretive tendencies. They can struggle with manipulative behavior and distrust. This remedy can help address their need for control and the fear of vulnerability.

Nux Vomica Suits those who are self-destructive and vindictive. They can exhibit intense behavior and hold grudges. This remedy can help address their fear of betrayal and the need for control.

Sepia Individuals may struggle with deep emotional wounds and fear of vulnerability. They can have difficulty forgiving and exhibit secretive tendencies. This remedy can help address their desire for power and control.

Staphysagria Suits those who tend to be self-destructive and hold grudges. They can exhibit intense behavior and manipulative tendencies. This remedy can help address their fear of vulnerability and the need for control.

Challenging Characteristics of Sagittarius:

Restlessness, Impulsiveness, Overconfidence, Tendency to exaggerate, Impatient, Lack of commitment, Difficulty focusing, Excessive idealism, Tendency to be blunt to the point of disrespect, Overemphasis on freedom, Disregard for details, Restlessness, Difficulty sticking to plans, Tendency to escape responsibilities, Tactlessness, Impulsive decision-making, Recklessness, Inconsistent follow-through, Tendency to overindulge, Impatience with routine.

Homeopathic Remedies for Sagittarius Characteristics:

Nux Vomica Individuals may exhibit restlessness and impatience. They can struggle with impulsiveness and lack of commitment. This remedy can help address their tendency to exaggerate and the difficulty in sticking to plans.

Pulsatilla Suits those who have difficulty focusing and lack commitment. They can exhibit restlessness and impulsiveness. This remedy can help address their tendency to escape responsibilities and the overemphasis on freedom.

Sulfur Individuals may struggle with restlessness and lack of commitment. They can exhibit impatience and disregard for details. This remedy can help address their tendency to overindulge and the difficulty of sticking to plans.

Lycopodium Suits those with impulsiveness and a tendency to exaggerate. They can struggle with impatience and lack of commitment. This remedy can help address their tactlessness and the overemphasis on freedom.

Challenging Characteristics of Capricorn

Perfectionism, workaholic tendencies, Pessimism, Excessive focus on status and reputation, Fear of failure, Suppression of emotions, Difficulty seeking help, Rigid and discipline, Difficulty expressing vulnerability, Cynicism, Prone to depression, Overemphasis on material success, Difficulty relaxing, Harsh self-criticism, Aloofness, Difficulty embracing change, Over-responsibility, Ambition leading to burnout, Excessive self-control.

Homeopathic remedies for the above characteristics.

Aurum metallicum (Gold): This remedy is often indicated for those who are ambitious, focused on success, and prone to deep depression if they feel they've failed. It's also useful for individuals who suppress their emotions and fear failure.

Calcarea carbonica (Calcium carbonate): Useful for individuals who are hardworking, diligent, and who fear change. These individuals can also be over-responsible and have difficulty relaxing.

Nux vomica: Indicated for workaholic individuals who are very ambitious. They can be excessively competitive, prone to burnout, and have difficulty relaxing. They may also be very critical and irritable.

Silicea (Silica): Perfectionistic people fear failure and are very rigid in their ways. They may also tend to suppress their emotions.

Kali carbonicum (Potassium carbonate): Helpful for individuals who are rigid in their routines and disciplines and can be overly responsible.

Staphysagria: Often used for those who suppress emotions, especially after feeling humiliated or embarrassed. It's also useful for individuals who have difficulty expressing vulnerability.

Natrum muriaticum (Common salt): This remedy is for those who have a hard time expressing their emotions and may keep feelings bottled up, leading to aloofness or feelings of isolation.

Arsenicum album: This remedy can be helpful for those who are anxious about their security, overly concerned with order and perfection, and can be very critical.

Lycopodium (Club moss): Useful for those overly concerned with reputation and fear of failure. They may put on a brave front but internally feel insecure.

Challenging Characteristics of Sagittarius

Restlessness, Impulsiveness, Overconfidence, Tendency to exaggerate, Impatient, Lack of commitment, Difficulty focusing, Excessive idealism, Tendency to be blunt to the point of disrespect, Overemphasis on freedom, Disregard for details, Restlessness, Difficulty sticking to plans, Tendency to escape responsibilities, Tactlessness, Impulsive decision-making, Recklessness, Inconsistent follow-through, Tendency to overindulge, Impatience with routine.

Homeopathic Remedies for Sagittarius Characteristics

Nux Vomica: Addressing restlessness and impatience, this remedy helps manage impulsiveness and commitment issues while reducing exaggeration tendencies.

Pulsatilla: Suitable for those with focus and commitment difficulties, Pulsatilla aids in managing restlessness and impulsiveness, promoting responsibility.

Sulphur: For individuals struggling with restlessness and commitment, Sulphur supports addressing impatience and enhancing attention to detail.

Lycopodium: Matching impulsiveness and exaggeration tendencies, Lycopodium encourages commitment and manages impatience, promoting more thoughtful communication.

Homeopathic Remedies for Capricorn Characteristics:

Natrum Muriaticum: This remedy addresses suppressed emotions, pessimism, isolation, and materialism. It can help individuals find emotional balance and connect with others more openly.

Arsenicum Album: For those who are over-workaholics, struggle with pessimism, and fear failure. This remedy aids in managing their ambition and perfectionism tendencies.

Lycopodium: Helpful for individuals with pessimism and over-workaholic tendencies. It supports self-compassion and eases harsh self-criticism.

Calcarea Carbonica: For those isolating themselves from fear of failure. This remedy helps balance work and relaxation, reducing rigid discipline.

Pulsatilla: Addressing suppressed emotions and isolation, this remedy encourages vulnerability and seeking help, thus diminishing the fear of showing weakness.

Sepia: Managing over-responsibility and resistance to change, Sepia promotes emotional flexibility and reduces the fear of displaying vulnerability.

Nux Vomica: For over-workaholics prone to isolation, Nux Vomica helps release excessive self-control and fear of failure, promoting healthier work-life boundaries.

Causticum: Addressing suppressed emotions and pessimism, this remedy encourages adaptability and openness to change.

Challenging Characteristics of Aquarius:

Aloofness, Emotional detachment, Difficulty connecting personally, Intellectual arrogance, Eccentric behavior, Rebellion, Conformity struggles, Emotional distance, Isolation, struggles with intimacy, Idea-centric, Impersonal communication, Disregard for tradition, Unpredictability, Difficulty expressing feelings, Over-independence, Stubbornness, Fixed opinions, Difficulty forming relationships, Emotional vulnerability rejection.

Homeopathic Remedies for Aquarius Characteristics:

Lachesis: Addressing aloofness and emotional detachment, Lachesis supports forming deep connections and emotional openness.

Pulsatilla: For those struggling with personal connection and emotional detachment, Pulsatilla encourages expressing feelings and seeking emotional support.

Phosphorus: This remedy addresses emotional distance and eccentric behavior, promoting balanced emotional expression and a stronger sense of self.

Nux Vomica: Addressing conformity struggles and intellectual arrogance, Nux Vomica encourages cooperation and openness to diverse perspectives.

Sepia: For individuals isolating themselves emotionally, Sepia promotes forming more profound relationships and embracing emotional connection.

Lycopodium: Supporting personal connection and emotional detachment, Lycopodium helps manage stubbornness and encourages open-mindedness.

Natrum Muriaticum: This remedy assists in expressing feelings and addressing emotional detachment, helping Aquarius individuals find emotional balance.

Silicea: Addressing aloofness and emotional isolation, Silicea promotes forming meaningful relationships and connecting personally.

Challenging Characteristics of Pisces:

Escapism, Impractical idealism, Over-emotionality, Vulnerability to influences, Boundary difficulties, Martyr tendencies, Gullibility, Reality-illusion confusion, Lack of direction, Self-sabotage, Victim mentality, Excessive empathy, Addiction proneness, Confrontation avoidance, Saying no difficulty, Overemphasis on emotional connection, People-pleasing, Assertion challenges, Losing oneself in others.

Homeopathic Remedies for Pisces Characteristics:

Natrum Muriaticum: Addressing escapism and boundary difficulties, Natrum Muriaticum aids in establishing healthy emotional boundaries and reducing vulnerability.

Lycopodium: For those with impractical idealism and over-emotionality, Lycopodium encourages finding practical direction and emotional balance.

Ignatia: Addressing victim mentality and excessive empathy, Ignatia supports inner strength and self-empowerment.

Pulsatilla: For individuals avoiding confrontation and being overly emotional, Pulsatilla promotes setting healthy boundaries and finding dynamic equilibrium.

Phosphorus: This remedy addresses escapism and losing oneself in others, helping individuals establish their identity and find their path.

Nux Vomica: Addressing confrontation avoidance and people-pleasing tendencies, Nux Vomica supports asserting oneself and building self-confidence.

Sepia: For those struggling with assertion and vulnerability, Sepia encourages embracing personal strength and emotional balance.

Lachesis: Addressing vulnerability and emotional sensitivity, Lachesis aids in finding clarity amidst emotional confusion and fostering self-assuredness.

In conclusion, a very well-trained astrologer, who is also familiar with homeopathic remedies, could look at individual astrology, i.e., natal chart, for instance, and gauge if a particular planet or planets are challenged and then refer to the the above information, and through a complete analysis of an individual symptomology, could prescribe a remedy to alleviate the condition. The same would apply to a challenged sign in one's chart, and the same procedure could apply to those characteristics used on the planets.

The Synergy of Astrology and Homeopathy: A Holistic Approach to Healing

In the realm of holistic medicine, the integration of various modalities has always been a subject of exploration and innovation. While classical homeopathic case-taking has long been a cornerstone of personalized treatment, there's an intriguing avenue to consider – incorporating astrological insights. This marriage of two ancient disciplines can amplify patient well-being and offer a more comprehensive understanding of individual health journeys.

Astrology, with its profound understanding of celestial bodies and their influences on human life, has been a guide for ages. By examining the positions of significant planets within different signs, we glean insights into a person's predispositions and tendencies. This astrological foundation can be a valuable adjunct to traditional homeopathic case-taking, enriching our comprehension of patients' inner dynamics.

The essence of this approach lies in studying the planets' placements and interactions. By identifying significant planets in different signs, we unravel the unique tapestry of an individual's constitution. The energetic interplay between planets and signs gives rise to diverse qualities, which, when examined alongside the homeopathic framework, can offer deeper insights into the patient's constitution and potential susceptibilities.

Central to this exploration is examining planetary aspects, especially the challenging ones. Just as in homeopathy, we aim to address imbalances, so too do we seek to identify potential energetic disharmonies in the celestial patterns. The intricate dance of these planetary energies, when combined with homeopathic principles, provides a comprehensive understanding of a person's mental, emotional, and physical landscape.

For instance, the Sun's placement in a specific sign can illuminate core vitality and self-expression. Paired with homeopathy, this insight offers avenues for addressing health issues related to identity and self-image. Similarly, the Moon's position in a sign reveals emotional nuances, which, when integrated with homeopathy, can guide treatments for emotional well-being and balance.

Of course, such an approach doesn't negate the significance of traditional homeopathic methods; rather, it complements them. Astrology acts as a complementary layer that enhances our ability to perceive the subtle dimensions of the patient's being. By tapping into celestial energies, we deepen our understanding of the individual's holistic state.

However, it's essential to maintain a pragmatic perspective. This synthesis of astrology and homeopathy is not intended as medical advice. It's a tool for reflection, exploring the interconnectedness of cosmic and human energies. Anyone experiencing health issues should consult a licensed healthcare practitioner for proper guidance.

In conclusion, integrating astrology into classical homeopathic case-taking offers a dynamic approach to patient care. By delving into the planets' positions, aspects, and their energetic interplay, we create a richer tapestry of understanding. This harmonious synergy enhances our capacity to address patients' needs holistically, acknowledging the intricate dance between the celestial and the human. As we embark on this journey of exploration, let us remember that healing is a multidimensional endeavor, and every layer we uncover brings us closer to the heart of well-being.

This synergy allows him to intuitively respond to external stimuli and challenges with courage and determination. His inspirational insights align with his proactive approach, making him effective in both understanding and navigating the dynamics of his environment.

What follows is a sample analysis of an individual's chart using both homeopathic, standard practitioners, methodology, and astrological insights:

Jane Natal Chart Interpretation: An In-Depth Scholarly Analysis with some recommendations of homeopathic remedies.

Planetary Placements:

Sun in Aquarius in the 4th House

Jane's Sun in Aquarius within the 4th house elucidates her propensity for innovation and originality, extending even to home and family. The unconventional disposition inherent to Aquarius aligns harmoniously with her futuristic outlook, potentially leading to a domicile replete with cutting-edge technology or a familial structure that diverges from conventional norms.

Moon in Leo in the 10th House

The Moon's placement in Leo within the 10th house illuminates Jane's profound emotional entwinement with her career and public standing. Leo's predilection for dramatism and leadership intimates a possible penchant for vocations that thrust her into the spotlight, where her emotional expressions find a public stage.

Mercury in Capricorn in the 3rd House

Communication Jane assumes a pragmatic and authoritative demeanor due to Mercury's position in Capricorn within the 3rd house. Her speech exhibits measured precision, reflecting her predilection for calculated articulation. This measured approach ensures that her words bear weight and garner respect.

Venus in Pisces in the 5th House

Jane's romantic inclinations are imbued with dreamy idealism, a characteristic stemming from Venus's placement in Pisces within the 5th house. Her amorous perceptions lean toward the ethereal, occasionally leading to the idealization of partners. This placement also suggests a profound affinity for the arts, potentially manifested as an ardent passion for transcendent forms of creativity, such as music or cinema.

Mars in Taurus in the 6th House

Occupying the 6th house, Mars in Taurus symbolizes Jane's embodiment of unwavering persistence within work and daily routines. Her vocational preferences may tend toward roles yielding palpable outcomes, possibly influenced by her appreciation for stability and her inherent aversion to change.

Beneficial Aspects:

Sun Trine Moon

The harmonious trine linking the Sun and Moon confers Jane an inherent understanding between her authentic self and emotional realm. This alignment facilitates a natural comprehension of her sentiments, allowing her to communicate her emotions with authenticity and ease.

Mercury Sextile Venus

The sextile aspect uniting Mercury and Venus embellishes Jane's verbal expressions with charm and elegance. This felicitous configuration endows her with the ability to articulate amorous sentiments and words of gratitude with eloquence and grace.

Mars Trine Pluto (in Virgo in the 9th House)

The trine between Mars and Pluto denotes a formidable drive and ambition within Jane's character. Her actions often stem from profound insights and transformative aspirations, potentially propelling her toward explorations of great depth or transformative journeys.

Challenging Aspects:

Sun Square Mars:

The square aspect between the Sun and Mars unveils potential conflicts between Jane's ambitions and her core identity. Striving assertively without overshadowing her intrinsic nature might pose a persistent challenge.

Venus Opposite Saturn (in Virgo in the 9th House):

The opposition between Venus and Saturn exposes Jane to the intersection of romantic aspirations with pragmatic realities. Lessons in love may illuminate the significance of patience and commitment even in the face of reality's constraints.

Moon Quincunx Neptune (in Scorpio in the 7th House):

The quincunx aspect between the Moon and Neptune underscores the difficulty distinguishing fantasy from reality within intimate relationships. Jane's emotional experiences may occasionally become ensnared by illusions or misconceptions concerning her partners.

Homeopathic Suggestions for Challenging Aspects:

For Sun Square Mars:

- Chamomilla: To soothe periods of heightened agitation or aggression.

For Venus Opposite Saturn:

- Baryta Carbonica: When feelings of love's restriction or delay become overwhelming.

For Moon Quincunx Neptune:

- Ignatia: To anchor Jane during emotional confusion or when reality appears elusive.

Additional Homeopathic Remedies for Challenging Aspects:

For Sun Square Mars:

- Staphysagria: To address suppressed anger and irritability, fostering healthier outlets for assertion.

- Lycopodium: Beneficial for enhancing self-confidence while preventing unnecessary conflict.

For Venus Opposite Saturn:

- Natrum Muriaticum: Addressing feelings of isolation and emotional constriction.

- Lachesis: For addressing jealousy and insecurities in relationships.

For Moon Quincunx Neptune:

- Nux Vomica: To promote emotional grounding and stability.

- Crocus Sativus: For addressing emotional fluctuations and maintaining partnership clarity.

Extended Insights:

The North Node's position in Sagittarius within the 8th house suggests Jane's life journey revolves around transformative experiences, potentially related to shared resources or profound spiritual revelations.

Chiron in Aries within the 11th house signifies potential wounds related to group dynamics. Her healing journey may entail asserting individuality within collective settings.

Black Moon Lilith in Cancer within the 2nd house implies struggles tied to self-worth and familial experiences, prompting her to assert her value more resolutely.

As one delves deeper into the intricate cosmic tapestry woven within Jane's natal chart, the scholarly perspective illuminates the complex interplay of planetary energies shaping her existence. This comprehensive analysis empowers her to navigate life's celestial currents with a profound understanding, guiding her journey with sagacity, poise, and an enriched knowledge of the cosmic symphony at play.

In Conclusion:

This culmination of exploration traverses the realms of astrology and homeopathic medicine, yielding a realization of profound importance. It is imperative to underline that this is no mere intellectual endeavor; instead, it encapsulates a substantive connection that bridges cosmic influences with the domain of well-being.

The intricate interplay we have dissected here transcends the realm of theoretical constructs. It signifies a dynamic symphony orchestrating the harmonious rhythms of the universe with the complex fabric of human health. Astrology emerges as the medium unveiling the patterns governing this cosmic ballet, thereby illuminating the profound impact of celestial bodies on human existence. In parallel, within the domain of homeopathy, these cosmic resonances find embodiment in the vibrational nuances of remedies.

Human beings, in essence, serve as conduits for energies, channeling frequencies that traverse the cosmos. The amalgamation of astrology with the framework of homeopathic medicine bridges the chasm that separates the celestial and the human, binding the macrocosmic and the microcosmic dimensions. This synthesis prompts the infusion of cosmic sagacity into the essence of daily living.

Remedies, in this intricate fusion, evolve into vessels of celestial insight. They acquire the archetypal attributes affiliated with planets and signs, resonating following the cosmic cadence that pervades the universe. Analogous to the lunar phases' cyclical progression, remedies mirror the pulsating rhythms of healing, recalibrating disharmonies, aligning energies, and invigorating vitality.

The synchronized synergy of astrology and homeopathy urges us to acknowledge our involvement in a grand narrative, where celestial, terrestrial, stars, planets, and human entities converge as interconnected threads within the fabric of existence. The birth chart assumes the role of a nautical chart, guiding individuals through the labyrinthine corridors of their health expedition. In tandem, remedies transform into guides, assisting in navigating the intricate landscape of well-being.

In traversing the passage of time, our forebears looked skyward, seeking guidance and warnings within the celestial bodies. Modernity, however, often distances us from these cosmic narratives. This alliance between astrology and homeopathy reminds us of our ongoing connection with the cosmos – a tether spanning millennia. It affirms that the universe's pulse beats within us, guiding our journey toward well-being.

Some Striking Similarities Between Astrology and Homeopathic Medicine

Astrology and homeopathy have roots in ancient systems of understanding and have been used for centuries to aid individuals in various aspects of their lives. While they have distinct practices and philosophies, they share some underlying themes and approaches.

Holistic Approach:

Astrology views the individual as a whole, taking into account not just the sun sign (which most people know as their 'zodiac sign') but the entire birth chart, which includes the positions of all the planets at the time of birth. Homeopathy treats the individual as a whole rather than just addressing specific symptoms. A homeopath considers emotional, mental, and physical aspects before recommending a remedy.

Individualized Treatment/Analysis:

Every person's natal chart in astrology is unique based on the time and place of their birth. Astrologers provide insights tailored to this personal chart. In homeopathy, remedies are chosen based on the person's symptoms, emotions, and general constitution. What works for one person may not necessarily work for another with the same ailment.

Energetic Influence:

Astrology believes in the influence of cosmic energies on individuals, with planetary positions affecting human disposition and events. Homeopathy operates on the principle of 'like cures like.' It's believed that the energetic essence of the substance, when highly diluted, can stimulate the body's healing process.

Nature's Connection:

Astrology relies on the natural cycles of celestial bodies and their positions in the cosmos. Homeopathy uses natural substances (plant, mineral, animal) as the basis for its remedies.

Ancient Roots:

Astrology has ancient roots in Babylonian, Egyptian, and Greco-Roman civilizations. While homeopathy is more modern than astrology, having been founded in the late 18th century by Samuel Hahnemann, it draws on ancient healing principles.

Pp

Intuitive and Empathetic Practice:

Practitioners in both fields often develop a deep sense of intuition and empathy. Astrologers 'read' a chart, looking for patterns and connections, while homeopaths 'read' a patient, considering even subtle emotional or mental signs.

Both astrology and homeopathy offer unique perspectives on understanding and aiding the human experience. They resonate with those who seek alternative or complementary paths to self-awareness and healing, emphasizing the interconnectedness of the individual with the world around them.

Microcosm and Macrocosm: Exploring the Age-Old Concept That Humans (Microcosm) Reflect the Larger Universe (Macrocosm)

The interplay between the microcosm and the macrocosm is a central theme that reverberated throughout the annals of philosophical, spiritual, and scientific thought. Rooted in ancient traditions, the idea suggests that individual human beings (the microcosm) reflect or are a miniature version of the larger universe or cosmos (the macrocosm). This principle echoes in both astrology and homeopathy, though in different ways. Let's delve into this profound connection:

The microcosm-macrocosm concept dates back to ancient civilizations. The Greeks, for instance, believed that the human body was a small universe in itself, mirroring the greater cosmos. Similarly, the old Chinese concept of Tao believes in cosmic harmony, where every individual element reflects its entirety.

Astrology operates on the foundational principle that the cosmos, or macrocosm, affects individual human lives, the microcosm. The positions and movements of celestial bodies at the time of one's birth are thought to shape their character, destiny, and life events.

Natal Charts: These are essentially cosmic snapshots of the universe at the moment of an individual's birth. They represent how the macrocosm (universe) at that time influences the microcosm (individual).

Transits: As planets move, they interact with the natal positions, suggesting that our microcosmic experiences continue to evolve in response to the changing macrocosmic patterns.

While homeopathy primarily focuses on the principle of 'like cures like,' some interpretations of its philosophy resonate with the microcosm-macrocosm relationship.

Vital Force: Homeopathy believes in a strong force or energy within every individual. This energy is a microcosmic reflection of the more incredible life force or significance of the universe.

Remedies: Derived from natural substances, these are believed to contain the essence or spirit of the source material, whether it's a plant, mineral, or animal. This essence mirrors the macrocosmic energies of nature within the microcosmic realm of the individual.

Both astrology and homeopathy, through their respective lenses, promote the idea of interconnectedness and unity between the individual and the universe.

Hermetic Philosophy: "As above, so below; as below, so above." This ancient Hermetic axiom beautifully encapsulates the microcosm-macrocosm relationship. Both astrology and homeopathy resonate with this, suggesting that by understanding one level (individual or cosmic), insights can be gained about the other.

If individuals are genuine reflections of the greater universe, then healing modalities like astrology and homeopathy offer pathways to balance and well-being by addressing physical symptoms and deeper cosmic connections.

Astrological Remediation: Astrologers often suggest remedies based on planetary positions to align individual energies with the cosmos.

Homeopathic Healing: Using remedies that resonate with an individual's vital force, homeopathy seeks to restore balance and harmony, mirroring the natural equilibrium of the cosmos.

In conclusion, the microcosm-macrocosm principle is a testament to humanity's perennial quest for connection and understanding. By viewing ourselves as unique entities and reflections of a grand cosmic design, we find avenues for deeper introspection, healing, and unity in the vast tapestry of existence.

Another interesting parallel between astrology and homeopathic medicine is the concept of holism.

Holism is the idea that systems and their properties should be viewed as wholes, not just as a collection of parts. This approach believes that an individual system (a human being, an ecosystem, or a social group) is more than just the sum of its parts. Instead, the system as a whole determines how its functions behave. It contrasts with reductionism, which aims to understand complex systems by reducing them to the interactions of their parts. The focus is on the interconnectedness and interdependence of all aspects of a system. Holism believes understanding the whole system can offer insights that aren't apparent when only studying individual parts.

Homeopathy is a system of medicine that views the individual as an integrated whole - encompassing mind, body, and spirit. Homeopathy doesn't just treat diseases; it treats individuals with specific disease patterns. Two people with the same illness might receive different treatments based on their symptoms, feelings, and experiences. A homeopath will consider a patient's mental and emotional symptoms, as well as physical ones. Homeopathy believes that the mind and body are intricately linked, and imbalances in one can affect the other. Central to homeopathy is the belief in a "vital force" or "life energy" that maintains health. Disease is seen as a disturbance of this vital force, and homeopathic remedies aim to restore balance.

Astrology studies the positions and movements of celestial bodies and their potential influence on human affairs and natural phenomena. An individual's natal chart, or birth chart, is a snapshot of the universe at the exact time of birth.

It represents the positions of the planets and other celestial bodies, and each interprets various aspects of the individual's personality, emotions, and potential life path. In astrology, each world, sign, and house is interconnected. The relationships between planets can indicate areas of tension, harmony, or focus on a person's life. Astrologers believe that as worlds continue to move and evolve, they interact with the positions of the planets in one's natal chart, indicating potential phases or challenges in life.

Astrology views individuals as being intrinsically linked to the cosmos. The positions and movements of celestial bodies are believed to mirror the internal rhythms and patterns of individuals and even societies.

Both homeopathy and astrology employ a holistic approach, emphasizing the interconnectedness of various elements, whether symptoms in the body or positions of celestial bodies. They prioritize understanding the individual or situation as a complete system rather than focusing solely on isolated parts.

Homeopathic medicine and Astrology also share an affinity for symbolism and interpretation.

Astrology is steeped in a rich tapestry of symbols that represent celestial bodies, their positions, and their relationships with one another. Every astrological element, from the zodiac signs to the planets and the houses, has its symbolic representation.

Planetary Symbols: Each planet symbolizes different facets of life. For instance, Venus represents love and beauty, while Mars signifies aggression and drive.

Zodiac Signs: The twelve zodiac signs, ranging from Aries to Pisces, are symbols representing inherent characteristics and traits. Each character has its logo, like the Lion for Leo or the Scorpion for Scorpio.

Houses: The twelve houses in an astrological chart symbolize different life areas, from self-image to relationships and careers.

Aspects: These are angles the planets form with each other and have their symbols. For example, the "trine" (120°) indicates harmony, while the "square" (90°) suggests tension.

In astrology, interpreting these symbols involves understanding their meanings and how they relate. Placing a planet in a specific sign or house and its aspects to other planets can provide insights into an individual's personality, tendencies, and potential life path.

Homeopathy is a medical system that interprets the subtle signs and symptoms of an individual to determine the most suitable remedy.

Symptom Symbols: In homeopathy, symptoms are symbols of the body's effort to heal itself. A cough, for instance, might be the body's way of expelling harmful substances.

Remedy Pictures: Each homeopathic remedy has a "picture" of many physical, emotional, and mental symptoms. This picture is created from proving, which is the testing of substances on healthy individuals to determine the symptoms they produce.

Miasms: These are inherited or acquired dispositions toward specific diseases or conditions. Samuel Hahnemann, the founder of homeopathy, described them as "infectious principles" or underlying causes of diseases. They have their symbols and interpretations, which can guide treatment.

Potency and Dose: The dilution and vigor of a remedy (its strength) are symbolically significant. Higher forces might be used for deeper, more chronic conditions, while lower potencies could be used for acute symptoms.

For a homeopath, interpreting these symbols means understanding the nuanced differences between remedies and matching the remedy picture to the patient's symptom profile. This is a meticulous process of observation, inquiry, and understanding of the subtle indications presented by the patient.

Both astrology and homeopathy are deeply symbolic practices that rely on interpreting these symbols to provide insights, whether into an individual's life path and personality or their health and well-being. While the characters might seem straightforward, their interpretation requires a depth of knowledge, understanding, and intuition. Both disciplines see the individual as a holistic entity, where signs and symptoms, or planetary placements, are interconnected pieces of a giant puzzle.

Both homeopathic medicine and astrology have some shared ancient roots. Although distinct, they often intersect in ancient medical practices and philosophical texts.

As we have witnessed, developed in the late 18th century by Samuel Hahnemann, its core principle is "like cures like," suggesting that a substance causing symptoms in a healthy person can treat similar symptoms in a sick person when given in the diluted form.

Much older, with origins tracing back to Babylonian times, astrology posits that celestial events influence human events and individual characteristics.

Both fields have deep historical connections to ancient medical practices:

The Greeks believed in the balance of the four humors (blood, phlegm, yellow bile, and black bile). The compensation or imbalance of these humors was thought to correlate with certain astrological events. For example, Mars, being hot and dry, was associated with yellow bile (choler).

Hippocrates, often called the father of medicine, is famously quoted as saying, "He who does not understand astrology is not a doctor but a fool."

Healing Through Individualized Resonance

Homeopathy, as a holistic therapeutic approach, sees symptoms not merely as problems to be eradicated but as manifestations of deeper imbalances within the individual.

Homeopaths adopt a comprehensive interview technique. They don't just focus on the ailment but dive deep into a person's emotional state, personal history, preferences (like food and temperature), and even seemingly unrelated physical symptoms. This vast array of information assists in sketching a holistic image of the person, ensuring the remedy resonates at every level.

The homeopathic Materia Medica is a compendium of remedies, each with its profile of symptoms and characteristics. A remedy isn't chosen solely because of a few matching signs but because its shape resonates with the totality of the individual's state. For instance, while multiple remedies might address headaches, the exact nature of the headache, accompanying symptoms, and emotional conditions help refine the choice.

Given the deep individualization intrinsic to both fields, it's perhaps unsurprising that there's been a convergence:

Some practitioners use astrological insights to refine their remedy choices. For instance, Saturn's influence might highlight deep-seated fears or chronic issues, pointing the homeopath towards remedies known for similar themes.

Both astrology and homeopathy operate from a philosophical standpoint that values the individual's nuanced experience. Rather than offering generic solutions, both disciplines respect the intricate interplay of factors shaping each person's life and health.

Astrology and homeopathic medicine, despite stemming from different paradigms, intersect beautifully in their profound respect for individuality. The intricate celestial dance at the moment of one's birth, much like the nuanced array of symptoms presented to a homeopath, tells a unique story. Both fields challenge the conventional, standardized approach to understanding humans, advocating for a richer, more intricate, and personalized understanding of each individual's journey.

Homeopathic remedies, on the other hand, are a system of alternative medicine that has been in use for over two centuries. Homeopathy considers the patient as a whole, addressing not just the physical symptoms but also the emotional and mental aspects. This comprehensive approach can lead to more profound healing. Since homeopathic remedies are highly diluted, many believe they offer treatments with minimal risks of side effects, making them a safer alternative for those who are sensitive to conventional medications. Homeopathy is based on the principle of "like cures." The idea is that substances that cause symptoms in healthy people can be used in diluted forms to stimulate the body's natural healing processes.

Some individuals with chronic conditions claim to find relief from their symptoms through homeopathic treatments when other modalities have failed. Some homeopathic remedies are geared towards treating emotional and psychological conditions, from anxiety and depression to trauma. Enthusiasts claim that these treatments can provide profound relief and promote mental well-being.

In summary, both astrological readings and homeopathic treatments offer a range of therapeutic and psychological benefits, as per their proponents. While the scientific community often approaches these fields skeptically, the personal experiences and testimonies of many individuals speak to their significance in various cultural and individual contexts. Whether it's finding one's path through the stars or seeking holistic healing from natural remedies, these practices continue to be a source of comfort, guidance, and healing for many around the world.

In general, multicultural societies have significantly profited from these disciplines.

Homeopathic medicine and astrology have held sway in various societies over the centuries, influencing everything from pop culture to significant historical events. The societal impacts of these practices, often shaped by shifting attitudes and historical contexts, offer a window into the complex interplay between belief systems and society at large.

Homeopathic medicine, born in the late eighteenth century, grew as an alternative to what was perceived as the aggressive, often harmful practices of mainstream medicine. As it gained traction, especially in Europe and the US, its societal implications became more pronounced:

In terms of pop culture, homeopathy's popularity has seen waves, with it being endorsed by celebrities and influencers at various points in history. The endorsement often leads to spikes in public interest and adoption.

Societally, homeopathy introduced the idea of individualized treatment. It emphasized treating patients holistically, considering emotional, mental, and physical aspects. This approach contrasted with mainstream medicine's more generic treatments, prompting broader discussions about patient care and individual needs.

Homeopathic hospitals and schools emerged in the 19th and early 20th centuries, signifying its institutional acceptance.

With the rise of big pharmaceutical companies in the 20th century, homeopathy faced challenges, often depicted as the underdog against 'Big Pharma.' This dynamic furthered debates on medical ethics, patient rights, and corporate influences on healthcare.

Astrology, with roots stretching back millennia, has seen its influence wax and wane across societies, but its mark on culture and history is undeniable:

Pop culture has embraced astrology wholeheartedly, especially in recent times. Horoscopes appear in daily newspapers, and "What's your sign?" has become a standard conversation starter. Social media platforms are rife with astrologers and enthusiasts sharing predictions, memes, and insights based on zodiac signs.

Historically, many leaders and monarchs relied on astrologers for guidance. For instance, Queen Elizabeth I had her court astrologer, John Dee, who played a role in selecting the coronation date. Such examples highlight astrology's influence on significant historical events and decisions.

Societally, astrology has often been a tool for introspection and self-understanding. Especially during times of societal upheaval or personal uncertainty, people have turned to astrology for clarity and guidance.

The division of time into months, the naming of days, and even the concept of the seven-day week in many cultures have astrological underpinnings, showing how deeply it's embedded in societal structures.

Regarding societal skepticism, astrology, like homeopathy, has faced its critics. The scientific community's challenges to its validity have sparked broader debates on belief, evidence-based understanding, and the role of intuition and spirituality in daily life.

In sum, homeopathic medicine and astrology have left indelible marks on society, shaping pop culture, influencing historical events, and prompting debates on broader philosophical and ethical issues. Their persistence and evolution underscore the human desire for healing, understanding, and connection to something more significant, whether it's the cosmos or the underlying principles of nature.

Modern-day relevance and the resurgence of interest in astrology in Homeopathy in the 21st century

The 21st century has witnessed a notable resurgence in the popularity of both astrology and homeopathy, with digital advances, social media platforms, and a global shift toward alternative healing playing pivotal roles.

The digital age, characterized by the ubiquitous presence of the internet and smartphones, has democratized access to information. This has brought astrology and homeopathy closer to individuals, breaking geographical and cultural boundaries:

Search engines and dedicated websites have made it easier for individuals to look up their horoscopes or research a homeopathic remedy. Instant access to information means that anyone, anywhere, can delve deep into these fields at their own pace and convenience.

Apps dedicated to astrology, such as Co—Star and The Pattern, provide personalized daily insights, making ancient art relevant and accessible to the tech-savvy generation. Similarly, homeopathic remedy finders and telehealth platforms connect users with homeopathic practitioners and resources.

Social media has played a significant role in the renewed interest:

Platforms like Instagram, Twitter, and TikTok are rife with astrologers and homeopathy enthusiasts sharing bite-sized information, testimonials, memes, and more. These platforms allow for community-building, where like-minded individuals can share experiences, ask questions, and learn from each other.

Influencers and celebrities openly discussing their experiences with astrology and homeopathy add a layer of mainstream acceptance and curiosity. When influential figures attribute their mental well-being or recovery to these fields, their vast followers often become intrigued and explore further.

The global move towards alternative healing modalities, underpinned by a growing skepticism of conventional medicine's one-size-fits-all approach and concerns about pharmaceutical side effects, has also contributed:

Many individuals are turning to holistic and individualized treatments, seeing them as more in tune with the body's natural rhythms and needs. Homeopathy, with its principle of treating the individual and not just the disease, fits seamlessly into this narrative.

The broader wellness movement, which encompasses everything from mindfulness meditation to organic eating, has created a conducive environment for both astrology and homeopathy. Astrology provides spiritual and psychological well-being, offering insights into one's character and purpose, while homeopathy promises physical and emotional balance without synthetic chemicals.

In conclusion, the 21st century's interconnected digital landscape, combined with a global shift towards individualized and holistic wellness, has breathed new life into astrology and homeopathy. These ancient practices, once relegated to the fringes, are now finding renewed relevance and acceptance in modern society, aided by technology and a changing global mindset. As people increasingly look inward for answers and outward for holistic solutions, astrology and homeopathy stand poised to cater to these evolving needs.

Conclusion

Many celebrities have embraced both astrology in Homeopathy and also the royal family, to name a few.

Katy Perry: The pop singer has often mentioned her belief in astrology. She once tweeted about Mercury being in retrograde, hinting at its potential influence on her life.

Megan Fox: The actress has shared in interviews that she consults with an astrologer and strongly believes in the spiritual world.

Madonna: The iconic pop star has shown interest in various esoteric fields, including astrology. She has referenced astrological signs in her music and spoken about the influence of astrology on her life in interviews.

Rihanna: The singer has tattoos of star signs and is known to have a keen interest in astrology. She's mentioned it in interviews and even integrated zodiac themes into her Fenty Beauty line.

Homeopathy and Alternative Medicines:

Paul McCartney: The former Beatle has been known to use homeopathic remedies and is a prominent advocate for vegetarianism and holistic health.

Gwyneth Paltrow: The actress and founder of Goop's lifestyle brand has been one of the most vocal celebrities promoting alternative health treatments, including homeopathy.

Cindy Crawford: The supermodel has publicly stated her use of homeopathic remedies for herself and her family.

Usain Bolt: The legendary sprinter used homeopathic remedies, specifically Arnica Montana, to help recover from injuries.

Jennifer Aniston: The famous actress is known to have used homeopathic remedies and is an advocate for various natural and holistic health approaches.

Orlando Bloom: The actor has spoken about using vitamins and homeopathic remedies to maintain his health.

David Beckham: The famous footballer used arnica to treat bruises and has shown his belief in homeopathy on various occasions.

Elle Macpherson: The supermodel has mentioned using homeopathic remedies to maintain her health and well-being.

Cher: The singer and actress has mentioned using homeopathy in various interviews and has credited some of her vitality to it.

Royal Family:

Queen Elizabeth II: The Queen is known to have been a patron of the Royal London Homeopathic Hospital, and it's been reported that she uses homeopathic remedies.

Prince Charles: An avid supporter of homeopathy, Prince Charles has been a vocal advocate for its integration into the National Health Service (NHS) in the UK. He has faced criticism for his stance but remains a steadfast supporter of alternative medicine.

Prince Philip: It's been reported that the Duke of Edinburgh has used homeopathic remedies, especially when traveling.

Princess Diana: Apart from her interest in astrology, the late princess was known to have used and endorsed homeopathic treatments.

The Royal Family's interest in homeopathy has been longstanding, spanning several generations. Their patronage and personal use have contributed to recognizing and accepting homeopathy in the UK and beyond.

These celebrities and members of the British royal court have significantly contributed to bringing astrology and homeopathy into the limelight, influencing the perspectives and choices of their followers and fans worldwide.

Future Outlooks:

Astrology:

As we gaze into the future of astrology, technology will undoubtedly play a monumental role in its evolution. The rapid advancements in AI and machine learning could lead to more personalized and accurate astrological readings, ensuring that the insights provided are tailored to each individual's unique astrological blueprint.

Online platforms, bolstered by ever-evolving computer software, will likely offer immersive astrological experiences. Augmented reality might allow individuals to visualize planetary alignments, facilitating a deeper understanding of their cosmic influences.

Evolving social views are likely to integrate astrology into daily life further. As younger generations, often more open to blending science and spirituality, come of age, the acceptance and practice of astrology could become more mainstream.

Research into astrology, once a field met with skepticism, might see renewed vigor. With improved computational capabilities, researchers could delve deeper into large datasets, exploring potential correlations between planetary movements and human behavior.

Homeopathy:

The future of homeopathy, much like astrology, is intricately tied to technological advancements. AI-driven platforms could assist in selecting the most apt remedy for an individual, considering many factors, from physical symptoms to emotional states.

Telemedicine, propelled by the ongoing digital revolution, is poised to make homeopathic care more accessible. Virtual consultations could become the norm, ensuring that individuals, irrespective of their location, can connect with renowned homeopaths worldwide.

Evolving social views, especially a shift towards holistic health and wellness, could further cement homeopathy's position in mainstream medicine. As concerns over the side effects of allopathic medications grow, more individuals might turn to homeopathy's gentle and individualized approach.

Research in homeopathy stands to benefit from advanced computer software and AI. These tools could assist in documenting and analyzing patterns in patient responses, leading to a better understanding of remedy effectiveness and, possibly, more acceptance within the broader medical community.

Conclusions:

Pondering the future trajectories of both astrology and homeopathy, it becomes evident that technology, especially AI and machine learning, will be pivotal. As the lines between conventional and alternative practices blur, thanks to evolving social views and robust research methodologies, both fields have immense potential to flourish in unprecedented ways. Their ancient wisdom, paired with modern innovations, promises a future where individuals have a more holistic and personalized approach to understanding themselves and attaining well-being.

As we venture deeper into astrology and homeopathic medicine, I invite you to join me on this captivating journey. These practices, rich in history and refined over centuries, offer insights and remedies that are as relevant today as ever. In upcoming chapters, we will delve intensively into these subjects, presenting detailed insights and perspectives for your consideration. Together, let's explore the art and practice of these intriguing fields.

As we draw this discourse to a close, it is incumbent upon us to internalize this awareness. The contemplation of the night sky should transcend the mere observation of distant celestial bodies;

it should serve as a reflective mirror that unveils the intricacies of human existence. Remedies should not be regarded solely as material substances; they encapsulate conduits that transmit the resonance of cosmic forces within their vibrational matrices. The cosmic ballet, far from being aloof, resonates profoundly within the depths of our being.

In the odyssey of healing, this awareness assumes the role of an abiding companion. Let us assimilate that we are composed of both stardust and human essence, existing as a harmonious confluence of the celestial and the terrestrial. This cosmic interplay, where ancient wisdom converges with the contemporary, yielding resonance, prompts us to assert, "Bring it home." This declaration invites the cosmos to partake in this harmonious dance, shedding light on our path and harmonizing our journey with the celestial symphony.

Chapter 6: Prospects of homeopathic medicine, and a summary of information.

In the final chapter, we discuss the developments and progress in the field of homeopathy and ponder its potential in the future of healthcare. We consider the growing interest in complementary medicines and how homeopathy is finding its place in mainstream healthcare. Additionally, we review ongoing research and advancement in homeopathic practices and continued efforts to establish the benefits of homeopathic medicine.

Principles of Homeopathic Medicine

Homeopathic medicine, introduced by Samuel Hahnemann in the late 18th century, rests upon a foundation of distinct principles that guide its philosophy and practice. At its core is the "Law of Similars," a principle suggesting that a substance capable of inducing specific symptoms in a healthy individual can be harnessed to treat analogous symptoms in an unwell person. This fundamental concept, known as "like cures like," is the cornerstone of homeopathic prescribing. By applying remedies that mimic the symptoms of the ailment, homeopathy aims to stimulate the body's innate healing response.

Central to homeopathy is the emphasis on individualization. This holistic approach acknowledges the multidimensional nature of each person, encompassing physical, emotional, and mental facets. Rather than viewing symptoms in isolation, homeopaths seek to grasp the interconnectedness of these aspects in understanding an individual's constitution. This comprehensive perspective allows for tailored treatment strategies that address not just the ailment's surface manifestations but also the underlying imbalances contributing to the condition.

Utilizing highly diluted remedies aligns with the "Minimum Dose" principle. This tenet posits that the therapeutic potency of a remedy increases as its dosage decreases. By employing minimal amounts of the active substance, homeopathy aims to engage the body's vital force, or life energy, without triggering adverse reactions. This delicate balance seeks to initiate a curative response while respecting the body's innate equilibrium.

Preparing homeopathic remedies involves a unique process known as "Potentization." This intricate method encompasses serial dilution and succussion, a rhythmic shaking process. The goal of potentization is to amplify the energetic essence of the original substance while mitigating any potential toxicity. This concept highlights the paradoxical nature of homeopathy, where increasing dilution is believed to enhance the remedy's potency.

Historical Development

The genesis of homeopathic medicine is attributed to Samuel Hahnemann, a visionary German physician, chemist, and linguist. Hahnemann's disillusionment with the harsh medical interventions of his era, such as bloodletting and purging, compelled him to seek alternative methods that were safer and more aligned with the body's healing mechanisms. His journey led him to discover the law of similars and the concept of potentization.

Hahnemann's magnum opus, "Organon of the Medical Art," published in 1810, is a pivotal milestone in the development of homeopathy. This seminal work not only codified the principles of homeopathic practice but also laid the groundwork for its emergence as a distinct medical approach. Within its pages, Hahnemann articulated his insights into the nature of disease, the role of symptoms, and the principles governing the administration of remedies.

Significance in the Healthcare Landscape

Homeopathic medicine occupies a vital niche within complementary and alternative medicine (CAM). Its gentleness, absence of invasiveness, and focus on holistic well-being make it an attractive option for individuals seeking treatments that align with the body's innate healing capacities.

In particular, homeopathy's individualized approach renders it a valuable tool for managing chronic conditions and ailments. In instances where conventional medicine might offer limited solutions or provoke undesirable side effects, homeopathy's personalized strategies address the root causes of illnesses, facilitating comprehensive and sustainable healing.

Although homeopathy has faced skepticism and debates surrounding its scientific basis, its popularity endures across diverse global cultures. Countries like India, France, Germany, Brazil, and the United Kingdom have embraced homeopathy as a therapeutic option. Countless individuals have attested to experiencing relief and improvement through homeopathic remedies.

Ongoing research endeavors continue to explore the mechanisms by which homeopathy exerts its effects and its clinical efficacy. While discussions persist within the medical community, proponents advocate for expanded recognition and investigation.

As society pivots toward integrative healthcare approaches emphasizing holistic well-being, homeopathy's enduring principles and personalized treatments are poised to contribute to the evolving healthcare landscape. This multifaceted discipline offers additional pathways to wellness, embracing the complexity of human health while aligning with the aspirations of those seeking comprehensive and individualized care.

The chapter that was dedicated to presenting a variety of homeopathic medicines under the title materia Medica can be helpful to many of the readers.

For Laypersons:

Gaining knowledge about the most commonly prescribed remedies in homeopathy becomes a powerful tool for laypersons, enabling them to navigate their health decisions confidently. This understanding goes beyond just recognizing the existence of homeopathy – it offers insights into the remarkable breadth of conditions that homeopathy can effectively address. As individuals become familiar with these remedies, they open themselves to healing possibilities that might have previously gone unnoticed.

This newfound awareness isn't just about theoretical knowledge; it translates into practical empowerment. With insights into frequently prescribed remedies, individuals can make informed decisions about their health journeys. Imagine having a foundational understanding of which therapies often alleviate specific symptoms or conditions. This knowledge, like a compass, guides individuals toward relevant options, offering a sense of control and participation in their well-being.

The utility of this knowledge extends further. It provides a toolkit for everyday situations where minor ailments and discomforts arise. Suddenly, individuals can tap into homeopathy as a form of self-care, addressing common concerns effectively and naturally. Imagine knowing which remedy might soothe a headache, ease indigestion, or alleviate stress. This familiarity empowers individuals to embrace self-help and first-aid solutions, promoting a sense of proactive health management.

The holistic essence of homeopathy is another dimension that unfolds through understanding commonly prescribed remedies. With this knowledge, laypersons can appreciate the intricate dance between their physical, emotional, and mental well-being. They start to see how a remedy doesn't just target a symptom in isolation; it engages with the individual. This holistic perspective aligns with the belief that health is a harmonious interplay of various facets, and remedies comprehensively address this complexity.

The allure of homeopathy lies in its gentle and natural approach to healing. With knowledge about commonly prescribed remedies, laypersons recognize they are exploring a path aligned with their desire for non-invasive and safe solutions. In a world often dominated by aggressive medical interventions, this realization can be reassuring and comforting. It fosters a connection with a form of healing that resonates with their values and preferences.

Integrating homeopathy with conventional medicine is a dynamic possibility that familiarity with frequently prescribed remedies can open up. Laypersons can learn to recognize scenarios where homeopathy can complement traditional medical approaches. This integrative understanding highlights the potential for a collaborative healthcare strategy, where diverse modalities work together to support complex health conditions. In essence, understanding commonly prescribed remedies paints a comprehensive picture of homeopathy's offerings, illuminating its potential as a holistic and collaborative approach to well-being.

For Homeopathic Practitioners:

Homeopathic practice becomes notably more efficient and effective when practitioners are well-versed in the 100 most prescribed remedies. This familiarity transforms the prescribing process into a streamlined and insightful endeavor. Practitioners can swiftly assess a patient's symptoms and constitution, mentally sifting through a repository of remedies to identify suitable options. The speed at which this happens enhances the practitioner's ability to provide timely and targeted treatments, a critical factor in patient care.

Beyond mere efficiency, understanding frequently prescribed remedies enables practitioners to embody the true essence of homeopathy – individualized treatment. With this knowledge, practitioners possess a palette of remedies to create customized solutions tailored to each patient's needs. This depth of personalization amplifies the potential for successful treatment outcomes, as it recognizes that health is a deeply personal journey influenced by myriad factors.

Familiarity with commonly prescribed remedies isn't just a marker of clinical expertise; it's a testament to a practitioner's commitment to their craft. The ability to navigate this body of knowledge reflects years of study, practice, and dedication. This depth of understanding instills confidence in patients, who often seek practitioners with a nuanced comprehension of remedies and their applications. It's not just about knowing the remedies; it's about embodying the spirit of homeopathic healing.

The compilation of frequently prescribed remedies serves as more than just a collection of insights; it's a trove of evidence that underscores the validity of homeopathy. By analyzing prescription patterns and observing the outcomes, practitioners contribute to the growth of evidence-based homeopathic practice. This empirical approach challenges skepticism and adds credibility to homeopathy within the broader healthcare landscape. It's a continuation of the tradition of inquiry and discovery that defines the evolution of medical modalities.

Ultimately, understanding the significance of commonly prescribed remedies transcends mere knowledge. It embodies the essence of homeopathy itself – a journey of empowerment, understanding, and healing. Whether for laypersons seeking to explore their health options or practitioners aiming to refine their craft, the chapter on materia medica serves as a gateway to a world of healing possibilities and insights.

Respect for the Body's Innate Healing Wisdom:

At the heart of homeopathy lies the profound respect for the body's innate healing wisdom. The Law of Similars, a fundamental principle of homeopathy, acknowledges the body's ability to recognize and counteract imbalances. Homeopathic remedies gently nudge the body's natural mechanisms, allowing it to restore harmony and equilibrium. This philosophy instills a sense of trust in the body's inherent healing capacities, aligning with the body-mind's intricate interconnectedness.

Holistic Perspective on Health:

Homeopathy's holistic perspective views individuals as dynamic entities composed of physical, emotional, and mental aspects. By addressing the whole person rather than isolated symptoms, homeopathy recognizes the interplay between these dimensions. This approach ensures that treatments resonate with an individual's well-being, promoting physical healing and emotional and mental equilibrium.

Enhancing the Mind-Body Connection:

Homeopathy underscores the intricate connection between the mind and body. Emotional and mental states are considered integral components of health. Homeopathic remedies take into account the dynamic background of an individual, recognizing how emotions can influence physical well-being. By nurturing emotional balance, homeopathy supports a more comprehensive and harmonious healing process.

Personalized and Patient-Centered Care:

Homeopathic practitioners excel in providing personalized care. Detailed consultations delve into an individual's unique experiences, preferences, and symptoms. This patient-centered approach acknowledges the individual's narrative and fosters a therapeutic alliance between practitioner and patient. Remedies are carefully selected based on an individual's symptoms, promoting tailored and effective treatment.

Safe and Non-Invasive Healing:

Homeopathic remedies are prepared through a meticulous process of dilution and succussion, resulting in highly diluted solutions. This makes them safe and non-invasive, suitable for individuals of all ages. The absence of harmful side effects or drug interactions ensures that homeopathy can seamlessly integrate with conventional treatments, enhancing overall well-being without posing additional risks.

Promotion of Self-Awareness and Empowerment:

Through its holistic approach and emphasis on understanding one's unique constitution, homeopathy encourages self-awareness and self-empowerment. Individuals become active participants in their healing journey, learning to recognize patterns, triggers, and imbalances. This empowerment extends beyond health, fostering a sense of agency in various aspects of life.

Contributing to a Balanced Healthcare Landscape:

Homeopathy complements conventional medicine by offering an alternative perspective rooted in balance and synergy. Its natural approach aligns with the growing interest in integrative and complementary therapies. By contributing to a balanced healthcare landscape, homeopathy enriches patient choices, ensuring a diversified range of healing modalities.

Catalyst for Mindful Living:

The holistic principles of homeopathy transcend healthcare, becoming catalysts for mindful living. The emphasis on interconnectedness and balance encourages individuals to adopt similar perspectives daily. This ripple effect extends to nutrition, exercise, stress management, and overall lifestyle choices, enhancing overall quality of life.

Cultivation of Compassionate Practitioners:

Homeopathic practitioners embody compassion and empathy. The patient-practitioner relationship is built on mutual respect, active listening, and understanding. This approach nurtures not only physical health but also emotional well-being. Practitioners serve as guides, partners, and sources of support in individuals' pursuit of optimal health.

Elevating the Healing Experience:

Homeopathy transcends physical healing, elevating the healing experience to encompass emotional, mental, and spiritual aspects. By embracing a holistic philosophy, individuals are offered a comprehensive roadmap to well-being. The journey becomes a transformative process that addresses the individual as a whole, enriching not only health but also personal growth and self-discovery.

In conclusion, homeopathy's multifaceted contribution to society from a holistic perspective is a tapestry of respect for the body's wisdom, holistic wellness, personalized care, and empowerment. This gentle yet potent modality aligns with the evolving health paradigm, bridging the gap between physical health and emotional harmony. By promoting self-awareness, fostering balance, and enhancing the mind-body connection, homeopathy serves as a beacon of holistic well-being in the modern healthcare landscape. Its impact radiates far beyond remedies, inspiring a more conscious, connected, and empowered approach to health and life.

Opportunities:

Personalized and Patient-Centered Care:

In an era where healthcare is shifting towards a more patient-centered approach, homeopathy is uniquely positioned to provide personalized care that addresses physical symptoms and emotional and mental well-being. As patients increasingly seek treatments that align with their values and preferences, homeopathy's individualized approach resonates well.

Complementary and Integrative Medicine:

Integrating complementary and alternative medicine (CAM) into mainstream healthcare is gaining traction. Homeopathy's compatibility with conventional treatments makes it a valuable asset in integrative healthcare models. Collaborative efforts between homeopathic practitioners and traditional healthcare providers can provide more comprehensive and holistic patient care.

Growing Research and Evidence:

The accumulation of scientific research in recent years has contributed to the evidence base supporting homeopathy. Continued research endeavors can shed light on its mechanisms of action, clinical efficacy, and potential applications. Collaborations between homeopathic practitioners, researchers, and academic institutions can further strengthen the body of evidence and enhance the credibility of homeopathy.

The global shift towards preventive care and wellness aligns well with homeopathy's philosophy of addressing underlying imbalances to prevent the development of chronic conditions. As people increasingly prioritize maintaining their health and well-being, homeopathy can significantly empower individuals to take proactive steps toward optimal health.

Advancements in Technology:

The digital age has opened up opportunities for homeopathy to expand its reach and impact. Online platforms, educational resources, and telemedicine options enable homeopathic practitioners to connect with patients from various geographic locations. Technological advancements also facilitate communication, education, and knowledge sharing within the homeopathic community.

Patient Empowerment and Engagement:

Homeopathy strongly emphasizes empowering patients to participate in their healing journey actively. With the rise of health literacy and patient engagement, individuals seek more involvement in their healthcare decisions. Homeopathy's patient-centered approach aligns well with this trend, fostering a sense of ownership and responsibility for one's health.

Global Reach:

The digital landscape enables homeopathy to transcend geographical boundaries. Practitioners can engage with a global audience through online platforms, webinars, and virtual consultations. This global reach facilitates cross-cultural learning, knowledge exchange, and the dissemination of information about homeopathy's benefits.

Strategies for Addressing Challenges:

Advocacy and Education:

Addressing misconceptions and enhancing public awareness of homeopathy's principles and benefits are pivotal. Advocacy efforts can include informative campaigns, workshops, and collaborations with healthcare organizations to provide accurate information to the public and healthcare professionals.

To strengthen its position within the healthcare landscape, homeopathy can continue to invest in rigorous research and evidence-based practice. Collaboration with academic institutions, research organizations, and funding bodies can contribute to expanding the evidence base supporting its efficacy.

Homeopathy can actively seek collaborations with conventional healthcare providers, bridging the gap between different modalities. Joint educational initiatives, interdisciplinary partnerships, and referral networks can facilitate integrated patient care and contribute to a more holistic approach.

Open communication between practitioners and patients is essential in building trust and addressing concerns. Homeopathic practitioners can engage in transparent discussions about the principles, mechanisms, and potential outcomes of homeopathic treatments to foster informed decision-making.

Initiating dialogues and collaborations with healthcare institutions, medical schools, and universities can promote a better understanding of homeopathy's value. Inclusion in academic curricula, research projects, and interdisciplinary healthcare teams can help integrate homeopathy into the broader healthcare system.

Establishing international networks and partnerships can facilitate knowledge exchange, research collaboration, and advocacy efforts on a global scale. Connecting with practitioners, researchers, and organizations from different regions can contribute to the growth and advancement of homeopathy.

In the evolving healthcare landscape, homeopathy faces challenges and opportunities that shape its role in providing holistic and individualized care. By embracing opportunities, addressing challenges, and adopting strategies that promote education, research, collaboration, and patient empowerment, homeopathy can continue to shine as a valuable and empowering healing modality. Its potential to contribute to personalized care, preventive health, and integrative medicine positions it as a beacon of hope for individuals seeking holistic well-being.

Enclosing, I hope the reader gained a greater sense of control of their health. I intended to provide a sound basis to incorporate suitable wellness methods. I hope all of you feel a sense of empowerment over your lives, with your family, your children, and your community.

I wish all of us a wonderful life filled with joy, happiness, and good health.

Be well always.

Blessings.

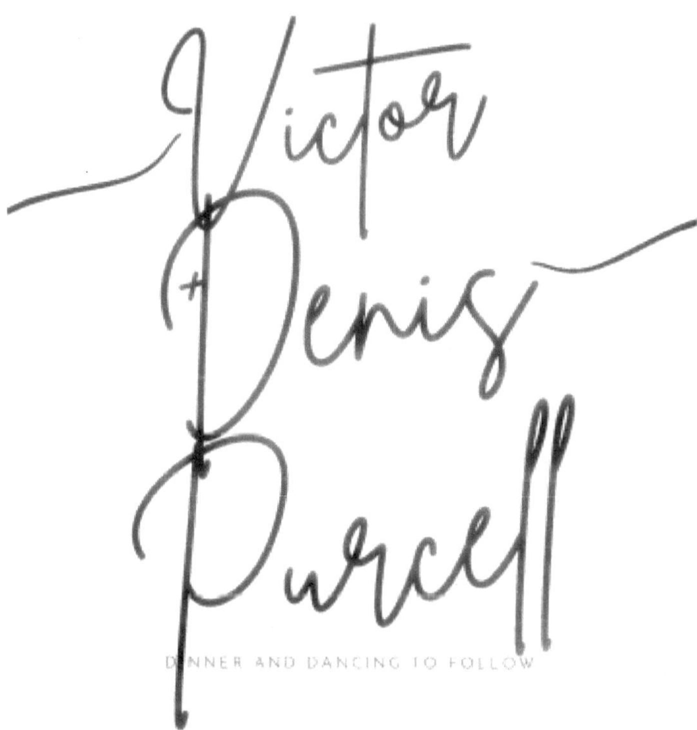

Dr Victor Denis Purcell

Below are some resources you may find helpful

."Organon of Medicine" by Samuel Hahnemann - This is the foundational text and primary work of Hahnemann, the founder of homeopathy.

. "The Complete Homeopathy Handbook" by Miranda Castro - A comprehensive guide to homeopathic remedies and their applications for various health conditions.

"Desktop Guide to Keynotes and Confirmatory Symptoms" by Roger Morrison and Nancy Herrick - This book helps identify the characteristic symptoms of different remedies.

. "Materia Medica Pura" by Samuel Hahnemann - This classic work describes various homeopathic remedies.

"Homeopathic Medicine at Home" by Maesimund B. Panos and Jane Heimlich - A practical guide for using homeopathy in common ailments and first-aid situations.

. "The Science of Homeopathy" by George Vithoulkas is a book that delves into the principles and philosophy of homeopathy.

. "Kent's Repertory of the Homeopathic Materia Medica" by James Tyler Kent - A widely used repertory that helps find homeopathic remedies based on symptoms.

"Lectures on Homeopathic Philosophy" by James Tyler Kent - A collection of lectures that explain the fundamental principles of homeopathy.

"The Chronic Diseases: Their Peculiar Nature and Their Homeopathic Cure" by Samuel Hahnemann is an important work that explores the treatment of chronic diseases with homeopathy.

. "The Prescriber" by John Henry Clarke - A practical guide to prescribing homeopathic remedies based on specific symptoms.

:

"Essential Synthesis" by Frederik Schroyens - A comprehensive repertory that combines information from various homeopathic repertories.

. "The Science of Homeopathy" by George Vithoulkas is a classic work that explains the principles of homeopathy and its practical application.

. "Clinical Materia Medica" by E.A. Farrington - A detailed collection of clinical experiences with various homeopathic remedies.

"Homeopathic Drug Pictures" by M.L. Tyler - This book describes the mental and emotional characteristics of various homeopathic remedies.

"Principles and Practice of Homeopathy: The Therapeutic and Healing Process" by David Owen - A book exploring homeopathic prescribing and case management.

. "The Homeopathic Treatment of Small Animals" by Christopher Day - A guide to using homeopathy for treating pets and small animals.

"The Genius of Homeopathy: Lectures and Essays on Homeopathic Philosophy" by Stuart Close - A collection of lectures that delve into the philosophy and principles of homeopathy.

"The Homeopathic Miasms: A Modern View" by Ian Watson - This book explores the concept of miasms in homeopathy and their relevance to modern practice.

. "Homeopathy and Mental Health Care: Integrative Practice, Principles, and Research" by Christopher Johannes - A comprehensive book that examines the role of homeopathy in mental health care.

"Nature's Materia Medica" by Robin Murphy - A materia medica that provides information about the source, preparation, and indications of various homeopathic remedies.

Certainly! Here are some more books on homeopathy for you to explore:

"The Homeopathic Treatment of Children: Pediatric Constitutional Types" by Paul Herscu - A book that focuses on constitutional types in children and their homeopathic treatment.

. "Homeopathy: Beyond Flat Earth Medicine" by Timothy R. Dooley - A comprehensive guide that discusses homeopathic principles, case-taking, and remedy selection.

. "The Spirit of Homeopathic Medicines: Essential Insights to 300 Remedies" by Didier Grandgeorge is an insightful book that provides a deeper understanding of various homeopathic remedies.

"The Homeopathic Revolution: Why Famous People and Cultural Heroes Choose Homeopathy" by Dana Ullman - This book presents case studies of influential individuals who have used homeopathy.

. "Impossible Cure: The Promise of Homeopathy" by Amy L. Lansky - A personal account of a mother's journey into homeopathy and its impact on her son's health.

. "Prisma - The Arcana of Materia Medica Illuminated" by Frans Vermeulen - An extensive materia medica featuring vivid descriptions of remedies.

"The Twelve Tissue Remedies of Schussler" by Boericke and Dewey - A classic work on the use of Schussler's tissue salts as homeopathic remedies.

"A Homeopathic Love Story: The Story of Samuel and Melanie Hahnemann" by Rima Handley - A biography of Samuel Hahnemann and his wife Melanie, providing insights into their lives and contributions to homeopathy.

. "Lotus Materia Medica" by Robin Murphy - A materia medica with information on over 1200 homeopathic remedies.

"Homeopathy: Medicine for the New Millennium" by George Vithoulkas - A collection of lectures by George Vithoulkas, a prominent homeopath, sharing his insights on homeopathy's future.